END ARTHRITIS PAIN . .
TENDINITIS . . . BACK PA

Read abou

D0401794

- How magnets provide relief from dental pain, whiplash, and head injuries

- The effects of magnet therapy on post-surgical healing

- What magnets can do to ease symptoms of osteoporosis and osteoarthritis

Plus

- Chapters on exercise and nutrition—including special sections on vitamins and supplements

- The role of herbs to relieve pain and inflammation

TAKE THE PAIN OUT OF YOUR LIFE WITH—
THE PAIN RELIEF BREAKTHROUGH

Julian Whitaker, M.D., is the medical director of the Whitaker Wellness Institute and the author of *Reversing Heart Disease, Reversing Diabetes, Reversing Health Risks, Dr. Whitaker's Guide to Natural Healing, Is Heart Surgery Necessary?* and the bestselling *Shed Ten Years in Ten Weeks.* He is also the editor of *Dr. Julian Whitaker's Health & Healing,* one of the largest health-related newsletters in the world. **Brenda Adderly, M.H.A.**, is co-author of the *New York Times* #1 bestseller *The Arthritis Cure.* She is a senior executive at the Rand Corporation and has worked in HMO and managed-care consulting, as well as for the United States Public Health Services in the Department of Health and Human Services.

Also by Julian Whitaker, M.D.
Reversing Heart Disease
Reversing Diabetes
Reversing Health Risks
Dr. Whitaker's Guide to Natural Healing
Is Heart Surgery Necessary?
Shed Ten Years in Ten Weeks

Also by Brenda Adderly, M.H.A.
The Arthritis Cure
The Complete Guide to Pills
The Fat Blocker Diet

THE PAIN RELIEF BREAKTHROUGH

THE POWER OF MAGNETS
TO RELIEVE BACKACHES, ARTHRITIS,
MENSTRUAL CRAMPS, CARPAL TUNNEL SYNDROME,
SPORTS INJURIES, AND MORE

Julian Whitaker, M.D.
&
Brenda Adderly, M.H.A.

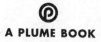

A PLUME BOOK

The material in this book is for informational purposes only. It is not intended to serve as a prescription for you, or to replace the advice of your doctor. Please discuss all aspects of your pain treatment with your physician. If you have any medical conditions, or are taking any prescriptions or nonprescription medications, see your physician before altering your treatment.

PLUME
Published by the Penguin Group
Penguin Putnam Inc., 375 Hudson Street, New York, New York 10014, U.S.A.
Penguin Books Ltd, 27 Wrights Lane, London W8 5TZ, England
Penguin Books Australia Ltd, Ringwood, Victoria, Australia
Penguin Books Canada Ltd, 10 Alcorn Avenue, Toronto, Ontario,
    Canada M4V 3B2
Penguin Books (N.Z.) Ltd, 182–190 Wairau Road, Auckland 10, New Zealand

Penguin Books Ltd, Registered Offices: Harmondsworth, Middlesex, England

Published by Plume, a member of Penguin Putnam Inc. This is an authorized reprint of a hardcover edition published by Little, Brown and Company, Inc. For information address Little, Brown and Company, Inc., 1271 Avenue of the Americas, New York, NY 10020.

First Plume Printing, May, 1999
10 9 8 7 6 5 4 3 2 1

Ⓟ REGISTERED TRADEMARK—MARCA REGISTRADA

ISBN 0-316-60193-4
ISBN 0-452-28088-5 (pbk.)
Library of Congress Card Number 97-76355

Printed in the United States of America
Design by Bruce Taylor Hamilton

CONTENTS

Introduction   3

Chapter One: WHAT EXACTLY *IS* MAGNETISM?   8

Chapter Two: THE HISTORY OF MAGNET THERAPY   21

Chapter Three: MAGNETS WORK   39

Chapter Four: PERMANENT MAGNETS ARE SAFE   63

Chapter Five: HOW MAGNET THERAPY WORKS   68

Chapter Six: MEDICATIONS: PAIN RELIEF   80
                  AT A PRICE

Chapter Seven: HOW TO USE MAGNETS TO TREAT   110
                  YOUR SPECIFIC PAIN

Chapter Eight: EXERCISE THAT HELPS, NOT HURTS   130

Chapter Nine: NUTRITIONAL HEALING: 147
                  YOU *FEEL* WHAT YOU EAT

Chapter Ten: TO SUPPLEMENT OR   163
                  NOT TO SUPPLEMENT

Chapter Eleven: PUTTING IT ALL TOGETHER: 180
                  THE FUTURE OF MAGNET THERAPY

Notes   185

Index   209

THE PAIN RELIEF BREAKTHROUGH

INTRODUCTION

This is the story of an extraordinary therapy that dramatically reduces, and sometimes entirely eliminates, many types of pain. It is
a therapy proven over centuries of actual practice that has begun
to take hold in mainstream America; it is utilized regularly in other
sophisticated countries (for example, it is used in a majority of all
Japanese households); and its efficacy is supported by documented
research. Even more important to you, it is a therapy that is "use-
tested" by any number of people, both unknown and famous. For
example . . .

   In 1996, Jim Colbert won $1.6 million on the senior profes-
sional golf tour. This was a new record, and it was his second year as
the tour's leading money-earner (in 1995, he earned $1.4 million).
The senior tour voted him Player of the Year. Not bad for a man
who, in 1994, had decided to retire from golf because he was virtually crippled by back and shoulder pain resulting from playing in 35
matches a year plus constant travel and practice. Magnet therapy re-
vived his career. (And according to the April 1997 issue of *Golf Magazine*, 90 percent of Senior PGA players now wear therapeutic magnets.)

   Dan Marino of the NFL's Miami Dolphins has stated publicly
that magnet therapy helped heal his fractured ankle more rapidly
while also reducing pain. The Dolphins' training staff is so impressed

by magnet therapy that soon the game bench will be covered with a magnetic pad.

Oscar-winning actor Anthony Hopkins, who continues to take on a variety of physically challenging roles, reports, "I suffered from terrible shoulder pain for years." Within a week or two of starting magnet therapy for pain relief, Hopkins was rejoicing that it "was the answer to my prayers."

Isolated cases? Not at all. They are merely examples of public statements by celebrities, widely reported in the media. Their statements are echoed by the private reports of vast numbers of people who have experienced similar pain relief.

Howard Eplin, James Canon, Arleigh Nielsen, and David Chestnut are long-distance truckers for the Indian River Transport Company in Winter Haven, Florida. Like many of their fellow drivers, all suffered from constant back pain. After using magnet therapy for two months, Howard Eplin found "great relief . . . a change from barely tolerable to light, or no, pain." James Canon reported more than "ninety percent of my pain has cleared." Arleigh Nielsen wrote, "My back pain is gone." And David Chestnut's pain, on a scale of 1 to 10 (10 being agonizing pain), fell from 9 to 1.

Note, too, the report by Joseph Kahn, PhD, an experienced physical therapist and a trained observer of pain syndromes, published in the *Physical Therapy Forum* of August 4, 1995. Kahn writes that his wife, Joyce, sustained an injury to her lower back (a strained sacroiliac joint) while moving heavy piles of sheet music, books, and musical paraphernalia. Muscle relaxants were prescribed, but were having little or no effect. While Kahn was able to give her some relief with twice-daily sessions involving ultrasound, massage, and other sophisticated therapies, the relief was not long-lasting. Walking remained difficult and sitting was a painful problem.

At this point Kahn attended a conference in Washington, D.C., and learned about the efficacy of magnets. Although basically skeptical, he nevertheless decided to try magnet therapy. After all, what did he and his wife have to lose? Kahn says that seconds after the magnet was strapped in place on Joyce's back, the pain disappeared. She remained pain free for several hours. When the magnet was removed, however, the pain returned, albeit at a much lower intensity than before. Subsequent use "provided immediate partial-to-full analgesia, permitting near-normal ambulation, and increased sitting time."

In 1974, Kyoichi Nakagawa, chief of Tokyo's Isuzu Hospital, distributed questionnaire sheets along with skin-patch magnetic devices to 11,648 persons suffering from what he described as stiffness of the shoulders, back, and neck, and headaches. More than 90 percent of those questioned reported the magnets to be effective.[1]

At any one time, an estimated 100 million Americans, about half the entire adult population, suffer from some form of chronic pain. Low back pain is so prevalent that one family practitioner in Gainesville, Florida, titled an article for *Hospital Practice* magazine "Death, Taxes, and Acute Low Back Pain."[2] In every industrialized country, back pain is the most common form of musculoskeletal ailment.[3] The American College of Emergency Physicians estimates that four out of five Americans will experience at least one episode of severe low back pain during their lifetime. According to the Back Pain Association of America, back pain is the number one reason for disability among people under the age of 45. In 1995, across the United States, the percentage of visits to the doctor for back pain was 73 percent in urban areas and 27 percent in rural areas, and each year the number of cases of failed back surgery ranges from 25,000 to 50,000.[4]

That's only one common kind of pain. More than 40 million Americans suffer from arthritis. We can't even guess how many women suffer from menstrual pain. Millions of people are also subject to frequent, often severe, headaches. Millions more suffer from bursitis, sciatica, and myriad other chronic-pain-causing conditions, including carpal tunnel syndrome. Quite possibly, you're one of the sufferers. If so, you certainly know how debilitating chronic pain really is.

In addition, almost everyone suffers from occasional pain following an injury or surgery; as a result of overexertion; or just from simple, but painful, stiffness stemming from everyday stress. It is no wonder that billions of dollars' worth of analgesics are swallowed annually in the United States: pain sufferers can easily spend $40 a month, or more, on pharmaceuticals.

Unfortunately, both over-the-counter and prescription pain-killers provide only temporary relief. If you suffer from chronic pain you know this only too well. You probably also know about the negative side effects that accompany the excessive use of painkillers. But, as most doctors will tell you, there is little else that can be done about chronic pain. Or, as one tough old lady explained to us as we were researching this book, "What can't be cured must be endured."

Well, in Germany, Japan, and many other countries around the world — and among the patients of a small but growing group of American physicians — there is something to be done beyond gritting one's teeth. Their approach to chronic pain is different: they seek to eliminate it!

Their treatment is not just effective, it is also exceedingly simple. *It is the application of a magnet (similar to a refrigerator magnet, only much stronger) to the sites that cause pain.*

As you read this book, you will see that members of the scientific community don't yet know everything about magnetic field therapy. Some suspect that magnets can help with many conditions besides pain, such as impotence, infections, and gastritis; others are skeptical. But two things about magnets are certain: They can lessen or eliminate many types of pain, and they are safe. And when coupled with a stress management plan, a diet and exercise program, and other traditional and/or complementary medical therapies as appropriate, the effectiveness of magnet therapy is often enhanced.

By the time you finish this book, we trust you will be an advocate for magnet therapy just as we are. For now, however, hold on to your skepticism; it's healthy! And let us start to convince you of the power of magnets by answering the most frequently asked questions associated with reducing and eliminating pain using therapeutic magnets.

Chapter One

WHAT EXACTLY *IS* MAGNETISM?

If you're looking for a simple, straightforward definition of magnetism, you may get a bit frustrated. Reference sources tend to send you into a useless tail-chase by defining magnetism as the force possessed by magnets, and defining magnets as pieces of metal that possess magnetism. Physicists and doctors who study and work with magnetic fields for a living seem to have an easier time *describing* where it comes from and how it behaves than saying simply *what it is*. Even sources targeted to the layperson, such as ordinary encyclopedias like Collier's, provide definitions of little value, such as "the force electric currents exert on other electric currents." The 1995 *Grolier Multimedia Encyclopedia* defines magnetism as "a general term that refers to the effects originating from the electromagnetic interactions of particles." Again, not very helpful, especially in the context of a discussion of permanent magnets, the focus of this book, because permanent magnets do not have an electric component.

Why is magnetism so hard to define beyond "it's what sticks the note to the fridge"? Perhaps it's because among the very basic building blocks of all matter and energy, magnetism is high up on the short list.

Scientists say that magnetism and electricity are closely related, and together make up one of the primary forces in the universe, called *electromagnetism*. Electric and magnetic fields are all around us, and while we may think of them as constituting an "electromagnetic force," individually they are different. An electric current flowing through a wire creates a magnetic field around the wire, whereas a magnet moving near a copper wire, for example, can induce an electric current in the wire. (See figures A and B.)

This was confirmed back in the 1800s, starting with Hans Christian Oersted, a Danish physicist and chemist, who in 1820 observed that an electric current flowing through a wire caused the needle of a magnetic compass to rotate, thus proving that magnets and electricity were related. Following that, French physicist André-Marie Ampère uncovered the mathematical relationship between electric current and the strength of a magnetic field. He subsequently proposed that it was the electric charge in atoms that caused magnetism. Then, in the 1830s Michael Faraday made his revolutionary discovery that a moving magnetic field induced an electric current in a coil of wire.

For thousands of years, scientists, doctors, healers, philosophers, and spiritualists have defined and explained magnets and

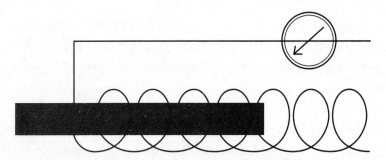

Figure A. The 19th-century British physicist Michael Faraday produced a steady current by moving a magnet into and out of a wire coil whose ends were joined over a compass. The current occurs only while the magnet is in motion.

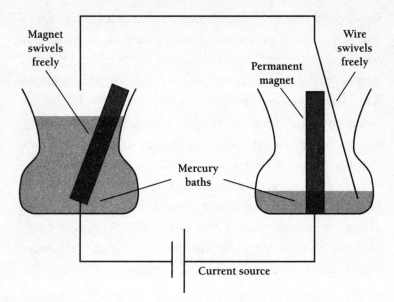

Figure B. When current flows in the circuit, the suspended magnet on the left rotates around the wire firmly fixed in a bowl of mercury (mercury is used because of its superconducting capability). The wire on the right rotates about a permanent magnet anchored in a bowl of mercury, showing the mechanical effects of electricity on magnets.

magnetic force in terms of how they behave and how they affect the things around them. And as you'll see later in this chapter, these definitions and explanations have evolved and expanded along with scientific advances.

It is still common to describe magnets and magnetism only in terms of their effects on iron, steel, or other ferrous (iron-containing) metals. For example, bar magnets have two poles; opposite magnetic poles attract each other while like (or same) poles repel; and certain metals become magnetic when they're in contact with a magnet. Certainly those are a few of the most readily observable and dramatic examples of magnetism. Yet modern research indicates that, as discussed below, all electrical impulses create a magnetic field. Since all substances on earth — including all living beings — possess electrical impulses, it follows that they are influenced by magnetic force.

As you might expect, some organisms are able to take greater advantage than others of the magnetism that surrounds everything on earth. For example, in 1975 the scientist Richard Blakemore discovered a type of bacteria that synthesizes magnetite from iron oxide crystals. (Magnetite, an iron oxide compound, is one of the most widespread and abundant minerals. The ancient Greeks were quite familiar with its naturally magnetic variety, lodestone.) The magnetite thus causes the bacteria to act like tiny magnets, resulting in their aligning themselves with the earth's magnetic field. Blakemore was able to prove this by viewing the bacteria under a powerful electron microscope. Since then, numerous species of fish, birds, bees, and sea turtles have been shown to have magnetite in their brain, which may help them navigate during migration and food-finding trips — especially when visual cues are absent.

In a series of remarkable experiments also conducted in the 1970s, researcher William Keeton showed that homing pigeons used the earth's magnetic field as part of their navigational arsenal. By attaching a tiny magnet to the pigeons' heads, he confused the birds totally, so that they scattered in all directions.

The ubiquity of magnetism has enormous implications for human health, since our nervous system and brain functions rely to a considerable extent on electrochemical impulses. In fact, many experts agree that the human body itself is an electromagnetic machine, and that magnetic energy quite probably activates the formation and division of cells. As a result, we are creatures guided in many respects by the electrical and magnetic impulses coursing through our brain and body.

Thus modern science is busily confirming what healers discovered centuries ago: The magnetic field isn't just "out there" in the earth and its magnets; *it's inside all of us as well.* Furthermore, the magnetism outside us — whether it's from natural or manufactured magnets or from the magnetic force of the earth itself — has a direct and profound influence on our health and well-being.

We'll describe magnetism a little more precisely before we proceed. No doubt you will recall, from your school days, illustrations of the lines of magnetic force surrounding a magnet. You may also remember your teacher demonstrating this pattern by pouring iron filings onto a sheet of paper and placing a magnet underneath it. The filings organized themselves into the pattern of the magnetic field.

ELECTROMAGNETS VS. PERMANENT MAGNETS

Throughout this book, two types of magnets will be discussed, electromagnets and permanent magnets. Electromagnets are magnets produced by electric currents flowing through a cylindrical coil of wire called a solenoid. When the electric current is discontinued, the solenoid loses its magnetism. Placing certain materials inside the solenoid, such as iron, increases the strength of the magnetic field, a breakthrough discovery made by British electrical engineer William Sturgeon, who in 1815 built the first practical electromagnet.

Permanent magnets, the primary focus of this book, are not produced by the flow of an electric current. Rather, their magnetic field is created by the motion of electrons in the atoms of the material that make up the magnet, such as iron or nickel, and thus keep their magnetism after they have been magnetized. Early permanent

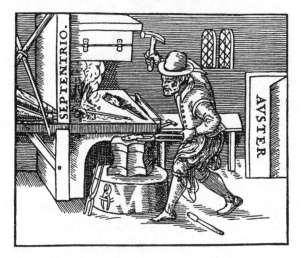

Figure C. Illustration from William Gilbert's 1600 edition of
De Magnete, showing how hot iron, when beaten and aligned
with the earth's magnetic force, can be made into a magnet.
(Septentrio refers to north, and Auster refers to south.)

magnets, aside from natural lodestone, were primarily made by forging carbon steel placed along the direction of the earth's magnetic field. (See figure C.)

Advances in 19th-century steel making led to stronger alloy magnets, which were surpassed in the 1930s by alnico products (magnets consisting of aluminum, nickel, cobalt, and iron), and later iron oxides containing barium or strontium. The most exciting advances were the subsequent introduction of rare-earth elements based on cobalt–samarium combinations, and the current "neo" magnets of iron, neodymium, and boron, which are 10 times more powerful than ferrite magnets and 100 times stronger than steel magnets made in the last century. Today, permanent magnets are manufactured by taking the elements in powdered form and pressing them under extreme heat in a magnetic field. The resulting mass, called sinter, is then magnetized in an intense magnetic field, a process that takes only a microsecond.

For our purposes, the differences between electromagnets and permanent magnets are (1) the magnetic field in electromagnets can be turned on and off, (2) electromagnets can be made to have more powerful magnetic fields than permanent magnets, and (3) magnetic fields emanating from permanent magnets are always static (motionless), whereas magnetic fields emanating from alternating-current electromagnets have magnetic fields that are always in motion.

With respect to pain therapy, it's sufficient to think of permanent magnets simply as those whose magnetic force is always present and constant. Individual permanent magnets differ in magnetic strength, but their magnetism cannot be turned on and off at will or "pulsed" electrically.

Let us here note a point of considerable importance throughout this book to make sure there is no misunderstanding. Both permanent and electromagnets have beneficial uses in modern medicine, and there is some indication that, to an extent, the mechanism by which they work is similar or at least comparable. Nevertheless, they are different. At a minimum, the vast amount of research (some of which we cite in chapter 3) proving the efficacy of pulsed electromagnetism assures us that magnetic fields constantly in motion produce biological effects. It doesn't prove definitively that static magnetism is equally effective, but circumstantially sheds much light on the efficacy of permanent magnets.

Pulsed electromagnetism, the process by which alternating electromagnetic fields are delivered in a time-varying manner, is widely used in hospitals and clinics worldwide to hasten healing of fractures, treat joint and muscle injuries, and for many other diagnostic purposes, such as conducting electrocardiograms, myograms, electroencephalograms, and magnetic resonance imaging (MRI). The equipment required for such electromagnetic treatment is relatively expensive and obviously not nearly as easy to use as is a simple permanent magnet. Proper application of the therapy requires special training. Apart from everything else, the therapy requires the patient to visit the hospital or clinic where the electromagnetic device is housed.

Thus, while there is much to be said for and about electromagnetic therapy — and we strongly endorse its use in hospitals under the auspices of trained specialists in appropriate conditions — the focus of this book is on permanent magnets because of their availability, affordability, and simplicity of use by any person in pain. Permanent magnets can last almost indefinitely if properly cared for. They are small, portable, inexpensive, and, by employing the techniques presented in this book, easy to use safely in your own home without special training. Above all, they work.

STRENGTH OF MAGNETS

The strength of a magnetic field is measured in units called *gauss*, named after the 19th-century German mathematician and physicist Carl Friedrich Gauss. The magnetic field at the earth's surface measures about 0.5 gauss, a standard refrigerator magnet (perhaps the most common form of permanent magnet) usually measures about 200 gauss, a certain therapeutic magnetic for treating neck pain marketed by a well-known company measures 2,450 gauss, and industrial-strength electromagnetic fields often measure more than 20,000 gauss. The gauss number represents the number of lines of magnetic force passing through an area of 1 square centimeter. Thus 500 gauss would mean that 500 lines of magnetic force are passing through the 1 square centimeter area.[1] But, to make matters a little more tangible, consider this: A 500-gauss magnet can lift an iron weight of approximately 2 pounds, and a 2,500-gauss magnet about 25 pounds.

How *much* magnetic field a magnet can have depends primarily on how much magnetic field it is capable of carrying. This quantity, known as its *saturation magnetization,* represents the ultimate magnetic field a magnet can produce, and varies based on the physical properties of the elements that make up the magnet. For a permanent magnet made of optimum materials, saturation magnetization is about 15,000 gauss.

How *permanent* a permanent magnet is depends on the materials' *coercivity.* Again, this is a physical property of the elements that make up the magnet. The higher the coercivity, the more permanent the magnet. The exciting advances in rare-earth elements have resulted in the manufacturing of magnets with dramatically improved coercivity. You may recall that magnets in the past were horseshoe shaped. (Many are still made in that shape today, but only for appearance purposes.) The reason for this was related to the principle of coercivity. Early steel magnets were of such low coercivity that the horseshoe shape proved to be the most efficient design, allowing both poles to contact the item to be lifted or moved.

As an increasing number of different magnet alloys became available, however, the ability of coercivity and saturation magnetization to measure permanent magnet strength proved to be too limited. Some magnets would have high saturation magnetization and low coercivity; others had just the opposite. There was simply no readily available index to offer usable comparisons. As a result, an index known as *maximum energy product* was developed. Its measurement is dependent on both coercivity *and* saturation magnetization. The higher the maximum energy product, the smaller the size of the magnet that may be needed. Thus, rest assured that even the tiniest of permanent magnets used to treat pain, such as the neodymium magnets, can pack a terrific magnetic-field punch. When shopping for therapeutic permanent magnets, be sure to compare the respective maximum energy products: it's commonly measured in units of *gauss-oersted* (GOe).

MAGNETIC FIELDS AND POLES

As stated, electromagnets create magnetic force when electric current passes through a solenoid. The field becomes stronger when the wire is wrapped around an iron rod. Up to a point (the saturation magnetization), applying more electric current and wrapping more coils of wire increases the solenoid's magnetic force. In an electromagnet, the magnetic strength is directly proportional to the strength of the electric current, so that the magnetic force ceases when the electricity is turned off.

When the flowing current is in one direction (DC), the magnetic field is steady, as is the field emanating from a permanent magnet. If the electricity flowing through the wire is alternating current (AC), then the rate of fluctuation of the magnetic field will be matched by the fluctuation of the electricity.

By contrast, in a permanent magnet the magnetic force is actually produced by the electrons that are spinning around the atoms of the material that make up the magnet, somewhat analogous to the electricity spinning around the iron core of an electromagnet. Each atom thus creates its own tiny magnetic field. However, an ordinary piece of iron, which obviously consists of many atoms, may not exhibit magnetism. The reason is that all magnetic fields, including those of individual atoms, have a direction, which we typically refer to as "north" and "south." (This designation is historical and has no particular significance except to define the direction of a magnetic field.) Iron atoms, unlike those of most other substances, can be ordered to all lie in the same direction. In a piece of iron that is acting as a magnet, many, or most, or sometimes all, of its atoms are lined up in the same direction so that they combine their individual magnetic fields to produce one large field. (See figure D.) If you hammer such a magnet vigorously, or drop it onto a hard floor, you may reduce or destroy its magnetism, because you are jostling the atoms out of alignment so that their individual fields again neutralize each other.

Iron and certain other metals are easier to magnetize because they have an abundance of electrons just waiting to get lined up, a feat possible when the metal is subjected to extreme heat. A number of nonmetallic substances have electrons available to do this as well,

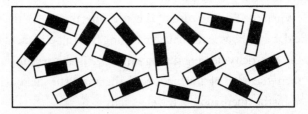

Figure D. Steel atoms have fully magnetized domains with random direction (above). Attaching a magnet causes them to point to the same direction (below).

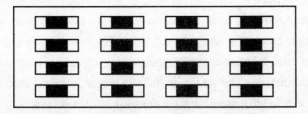

and completely organic magnets can now be made. (A common assumption is that magnetism is a property of metals per se; it is not.) These substances may have advantages over metals because they can be bent and shaped more readily and may be cheaper to produce, since extreme temperatures are not required.

Scientists believe that at various times in the earth's history — at approximately 200,000-year intervals — the magnetic north and south reversed themselves. This phenomenon was posited when 30,000-year-old rocks from an aboriginal campfire in Australia were observed to be magnetized in the opposite direction of the present poles. Subsequent study of successive layers of cooled volcanic lava flows that can be dated has enabled scientists to determine when reversals of the earth's magnetic fields have taken place.

The electrical currents flowing in our own bodies create magnetic fields that extend outward. The electrical currents flowing in our brains produce a magnetic field that can be measured by a device called a magnetoencephalograph, which produces a magnetoencephalogram (MEG).

Dr. Robert Becker notes in his book *Cross Currents* that we may be disconcerted to know that we, like all living things, are "surrounded by a magnetic field that extends out into space from our bodies, and that the fields from the brain reflect what is happening in the brain. The implications of this are enormous."[2]

Indeed they are! And not only in the context of seeking to learn more about the internal functions of the brain. For if we generate a magnetic field outside ourselves, it follows necessarily that the reverse also applies: magnetic fields generated by outside forces must be able to penetrate inside us and affect the electrical currents inside our bodies.

The earth's core of spinning, molten iron is credited with

turning the entire planet into one huge magnet, so that the earth is surrounded by its own magnetic field, which influences everything on, under, and above our planet's surface. Hence, every living thing on earth is wrapped in a natural biomagnetic blanket from birth to death. Research results are piling up that prove the importance of this force to our health. One example: Professor Holger Hannemann, in his book *Magnet Therapy,* reports experiments by Drs. J. H. Vandyk and M. H. Halpern for the U.S. space program in which they raised mice in specially prepared metal cages that would shield them from the earth's electromagnetism. Within weeks, the animals lost their fur and began to die, whereas animals raised in a normal environment remained healthy.[3]

Chapter Two

THE HISTORY OF MAGNET THERAPY

Centuries before the English term *magnetism* was coined, healers in China, India, and Egypt were using natural magnets to treat and cure a wide variety of human ailments. In ancient China, a system of medicine developed that still flourishes today, based on the notion that good health depends on the circulation of vital energy throughout the body via established pathways or channels, called meridians.

This internal life energy, known as *qi* (also called *ch'i* or *chi*), derives from two opposing influences or poles, yin (minus or negative polarity) and yang (positive). Illness results when the dual powers, yin and yang, are out of balance, the natural flow of *qi* is blocked, or when there is some disturbance in the normal symmetry between an individual's *qi* and analogous natural forces, namely the seasons and the five elements that were known at that time.

If you're familiar with modern acupuncture or acupressure, you probably recognize these terms and concepts. And you're probably aware that modern research is validating the ancient treatment techniques as medically sound and effective in blocking pain. Research scientists believe that is probably because inserting a metal needle into the skin generates a small electrical current, twirling the needle likely causes the current to pulse, and warming it may slightly increase the strength of the current. On the other hand, modern practitioners of the Chinese method of *qigong* massage now accept that the inner energy known as *qi* is, in fact, bioelectricity.[1]

As we will discuss later, some physicians believe that moving a part of your body through a static magnetic field may also generate tiny electric currents in the body much as some believe acupuncture does. At least one carefully controlled study suggests that, indeed, the two may be equally effective, although working in slightly different ways.

The ancient Egyptians clearly understood the concepts of polarity and balance, whether magnetic or not, and used them in their medical practice, ascribing a variety of therapeutic effects to lodestones. It is said that Queen Cleopatra, seeking to prevent aging, wore a lodestone on her forehead while she slept.

Not only the ancient Egyptians used magnets for therapeutic purposes, but also the ancient Arabs, Indians, Hebrews, Chinese, and Greeks. In fact, Aristotle is believed to have been the first in recorded history to speak of the therapeutic capabilities of magnets.[2]

Yet no matter how quaint, mystical, and obsolete the ancients' explanations of how and why magnets healed, the fact is that, just as with acupuncture, modern research is proving that they certainly knew what they were doing with magnet therapy all those centuries ago. Magnets could then, and can now, ease pain.

MAGNETS AND LODESTONES

The ancient Greeks were the first to use the word *magnet*. There are two different stories about how the term originated. In one version, attributed to Plato, a Greek shepherd named Magnes was tending his flock near Mount Ida when the nails in his sandals (or his iron-tipped staff) became attracted to a magnetic rock with such force that pulling free was difficult. If you doubt that story, the alternative, according to Euripides, is that the name was derived from Magnesia, an area in Greece rich in accumulations of iron-laden volcanic rock with magnetic properties, called magnesian stone. (In China, magnetic rocks were called *tzhu shih,* "loving stones," because of their ability to attract anything containing iron.[3]) Whatever the name's origin, throughout the centuries magnets have been used to relieve pain.

The name *lodestone* for natural magnetic rocks came later, with the invention of the navigational compass. *Lode* or *load* is derived from the Old English *lād,* which meant "way" or "course," hence, *lodestar* or "leading star," used by early sailors in navigation, and later, *lodestone* ("guiding stone") for the natural magnetic rock used in the compass.

PARACELSUS: BRINGING THERAPEUTIC MAGNETS OUT OF THE DARK AGES

We know from early historical writings that a popular treatment used by Roman physicians for arthritis and gout was the application of electric eels. It must have been a blessing for patients and doctors alike when medieval doctors began to use magnets to treat these inflammatory ailments, and others, including baldness. No doubt the magnets were considerably easier to handle!

The credit for bringing magnet therapy — and medicine in general — out of the Dark Ages goes to the great German alchemist, physician, and metallurgist Philippus Aureolus Theophrastus Bombast von Hohenheim. Born in Einsiedeln, Switzerland, in 1493, he later changed his name to Paracelsus (who can blame him?). Some say the new name was a way of acknowledging his intellectual debt to the great first-century Roman physician and writer Aulus Cornelius Celsus, who wrote one of the first medical works to be printed (in 1478). Knowing that Paracelsus was arrogant and conceited, and not well liked by his colleagues, others suspect he invented the name because it meant "superior to Celsus."

Modern "traditional" medicine, homeopathy, holistic healing, and magnet therapy all owe an intellectual debt to Paracelsus, who, after wandering through Europe in the early 1500s and being forced to leave the University of Basel because of his intellectual rebelliousness, finally settled in Salzburg, Austria.

Opposing the prevailing humoral theory of disease (that illness originated from imbalances *within* the body), Paracelsus began to teach and to practice under the guiding belief that some illnesses were caused by *external* agents and could be cured by specific remedies. By his advocacy of the use of mercury, lead, sulphur, iron, arsenic, copper sulphate, and other chemicals to combat these external disease-causing agents, Paracelsus became the first physician to establish the role of chemistry in medicine.

He was also the first to recognize the existence of a hereditary pattern in syphilis, to connect goiter with minerals in drinking water, and to observe that certain types of head injuries sometimes resulted in paralysis. He provided the basis for modern homeopathy by proposing that some diseases could be cured by minuscule doses of "similars," substances that could produce symptoms similar to those of the disease being treated.[4]

Going against much of the medical wisdom of the time, Paracelsus held a view akin to that of many ancient cultures about the relationship of people to heaven and earth, that there was some intangible life force in nature that could energize people. He thought it was internal, all-encompassing, and brought together the mind with the body; he named it *archaeus* (from the Greek word for "ancient"). Paracelsus believed it could indicate the state of a person's health and that illnesses could be treated by replenishing it through the natural energies found in certain herbs and foods. He thought magnets also had a power that could energize the body or replenish its energy, and influence the archaeus to promote self-healing.[5] Writings such as Paracelsus's *De origine morborum invisibulum* make it clear that he knew the earth is one gigantic magnet whose force permeates and affects everything on the planet.

It was already known that doctors and healers used magnets to retrieve pieces of knives and other iron parts imbedded in tissues; Paracelsus broadened the use of magnets to treat everything from the simplest diarrhea to various types of hemorrhage, and even epilepsy.

Indeed, we now know that all matter is magnetized or responds to magnetic force, although most materials are so weakly magnetic that their magnetism is not noticed in everyday life. Given sufficiently sensitive devices, physicists have been able to measure the magnetic properties of various minerals, glass, and, of course, living tissue. It has been determined that each person's body has varying magnetic energy characteristics that differ from person to person, and differ within the body as well. [6]

HEALING OR QUACKERY? EUROPE IN THE 1600s

By the 1600s, the medical use of magnets was something of a fad in Europe, for it tied in to the intellectual climate of an age when, as author Keith Thomas describes it, "the possibility of certain types of magic was a fundamental presupposition for most scientists."[7] So it's not surprising that in 1652 the British historian Elias Ashmole wrote, "If we should consider the operations of this magnet, there is no mystery, celestial, elemental or earthly, which can be too hard for our belief."[8]

William Gilbert, a mathematician and prosperous London

physician, was a harsh critic of those making claims about the extraordinary medicinal and spiritual powers of lodestones (one of which was that placing a lodestone under the bed of a sleeping woman would drive her out of bed if she was committing adultery), and debunked the use of lodestone salves and powders. Around 1600, Gilbert became a favorite of Queen Elizabeth I, as hardheaded a realist as history has ever produced, partly (according to some sources) because he was able to alleviate some of the by-then-elderly monarch's aches and pains. But she also supported him because she felt that his studies of magnetism for navigation might further contribute to her all-important naval supremacy.

Gilbert's major work, *De magnete, magneticisque corporibus, et de magno magnete tellure,* published in 1600, is considered by many to be the world's first great scientific treatise. In it, he proposed that the earth was actually a spherical magnet with magnetic poles near the geographical north and south poles.[9] A century later, in 1701, the English astronomer Edmund Halley would publish the first magnetic sea charts.

MESMER AND MAGNETISM

Just as he reached young manhood, the time was ripe for Franz Anton Mesmer to work his magic. One of the most famous and controversial figures of his day, Mesmer both vaulted magnet therapy into the public limelight and turned it into a sideshow. Born in Germany in 1734, Mesmer studied in Vienna under a Jesuit priest, Maximilian Hell, a highly respected astronomer and magnet therapy practitioner. Father Hell treated patients by applying newly developed powerful carbon-steel permanent magnets, bent into different shapes to correspond to various parts of the human frame, to their naked bodies.[10]

Mesmer, profoundly influenced by both Hell and the writings of Paracelsus, immersed himself in similar studies and practices. His doctoral thesis dealt with the influence of gravitational fields, planets, and cycles on human health. It proposed that a subtle "universal fluid," a kind of invisible magnetic energy, or gas, permeated the universe as well as all bodily fluids. The fluid had properties like those of a magnet, and an unequal distribution of it produced disease, Mesmer wrote; health could be attained by reestablishing the harmony of the magnetic fields within the body, which had different and opposite poles like magnets, thus rendering the human body responsive to the influence of the heavenly bodies. Accordingly, Mesmer used magnets to promote an "artificial tide" in the universal fluid and restore health to ailing persons.[11]

In his 1775 report *On the Medicinal Uses of the Magnet,* Mesmer described his cure of a patient who had previously uncontrollable seizures and other nervous system disorders by feeding her iron filings and then applying Hell's specially shaped magnets:

> [W]hen my patient had another attack, I fixed two magnets of horseshoe-shaped type to her feet and a heart-shaped magnet to her breast. Suddenly she felt a burning sensation spreading from her feet through all her joints like a glowing coal . . . and likewise from both sides of the breast to the crown of the head . . . the pains gradually went away, she became insensitive to the magnets. The symptoms disappeared and she recovered from the seizure.[12]

Certain that the cure had resulted from his influence upon, and control of, the flow of universal fluid, Mesmer began to refine and redefine the concept of magnetism. According to him, there were two types, animal and mineral. Animal magnetism was the natural force he observed in humans and other animals. It could be influenced by the magnetic force in iron or steel, which he referred to as mineral magnetism. Furthermore, the egocentric Mesmer believed he could magnetize just about any substance, living or not, by using his own particularly powerful animal magnetism; regular magnets could be used as conductors to "magnify" the flow of universal fluid from his body to that of the patient. Recent studies prove that Mesmer was on to something, even if he — like many pioneers past and present — was a bit like one of the blind men describing an elephant.

Mesmer outlined his theories in his *Memoire sur la discouverte du magnetisme animal* (Report on the Discovery of Animal Magnetism), published in 1779. He presented 27 theses or statements about his belief in animal magnetism and the use of magnets to treat illnesses. Thesis Number 23 stated, "From the practical rules I have established, it is clear that this principle [animal magnetism] can heal mental illness directly, and all other illnesses indirectly."

Indeed, Mesmer's own animal magnetism produced some seemingly miraculous cures. He restored the hearing of a deaf person simply by holding his hands over the man's ears. The persistent chest pains and stomach spasms of other persons disappeared when he stroked the areas. We know today that new medicines are more successful in their early days when doctors still have a passionate belief in their efficacy, so we can only assume that both Mesmer and his patients all had a powerful belief in the curative ability of this "new force" and its deliverer.

Mesmer traveled throughout Europe, enhancing his prominence as a healer wherever he went. He became so famous, in fact, that along with ridiculing the follies of romance, Mozart and his librettist Lorenzo Da Ponte paid tribute to Mesmer's influence on society in the 1790 opera *Così fan tutte*. Toward the end of the first act of the opera, two men pretend to ingest poison as part of a plot to test the loyalty of their fiancées. A maid speaks of a marvelous doctor who cures people without the use of pills or knives. Returning disguised as a doctor, she unveils a huge magnet from under her gown, touches the foreheads of the two men, and glides it along their bodies. Of course, they magically recover. While doing so, she sings, "Here is a piece of the magnetic mesmeric stone, discovered in Germany, made so famous in France."[13]

Controversy increasingly nipped at the heels of Mesmer's fame, however. In one famous case, he restored the sight of Maria Theresa von Paradis, an 18-year-old girl who had suddenly become blind at age 3. Admired for her musical talent, the girl was under the patronage of the Empress Maria Theresa.[14] Many famous and influential doctors had already tried and failed to cure her. Yet after Mesmer succeeded, the very same doctors who had observed and validated the healing reversed themselves and publicly declared him a fraud after the girl's blindness returned. (From our modern perspective, it seems that the blindness was psychosomatic and that Mesmer interrupted the blindness temporarily. And it certainly supports the view that he was adept at hypnosis, whether or not he intended to use the skill or was even aware of it.)

Furthermore, Mesmer surely, if unwittingly, fueled the fires of controversy through his own flair for the dramatic and his need to meet the rapidly increasing demands for his cures by treating more and more patients at once. Settling in Paris, Mesmer opened a healing salon where as many as 20 patients at a time sat around a wooden vat filled with water, iron filings, and protruding rods. Patients held on to the iron rods, through which the magnetic influence reached their bodies.[15] Sometimes a number of patients joined hands or were connected to each other by cords to facilitate the flow of the now-famous universal fluid. (One author has referred to this as the cornerstone for present-day group therapy.)[16]

"Assistant magnetizers" worked with Mesmer and provided instruction in the activities, which took place in a highly theatrical setting replete with mirrors, brightly colored fabrics and lights, and dramatic music, all designed to encourage successful therapeutic expectations. (Mesmer believed that mirrors and music intensified the communication of universal fluid.) Periodically the flamboyant Mesmer appeared in his elegant silk robe, carrying a glass rod, which he used, along with his hands, to coordinate and assist in the transfer of the animal magnetism he exuded.

Patients often appeared entranced, fainted, or would go into convulsions and then be taken to a recovery room. It was assumed that on awakening from these "hysterical fits," as one author referred to them, the person would be cured.[17] The patients were "mesmerized," and the word remains in our vocabulary today, occasionally as a synonym for hypnotized.

Given his outlandish behavior and many curative claims, it's easy to understand why many physicians and scientists considered Mesmer a showboating fraud. Still, he was the toast of Paris; ardent followers flocked to him for healings. Wealthy Parisians waited in long lines to partake of the experiences his fame promised. Among his supporters was the French statesman the Marquis de Lafayette, by then a Revolutionary War hero who sent letters to his friend George Washington commending Mesmer and singing the praises of animal magnetism.[18]

In an attempt to settle the controversy — and perhaps to stop the loss of their wealthy patients to the flamboyant Mesmer — opposing doctors and the French Academy of Science convinced

King Louis XVI in 1784 to establish an unbiased commission to determine once and for all whether Mesmer's treatment had any scientific validity. The panel included the astronomer Jean-Sylvain Bailly, who had computed the orbit for Halley's Comet, and the chemist Antoine-Laurent Lavoisier, who first demonstrated the role of oxygen in respiration and fire and is considered the founder of modern chemistry. Ironically for these two gentlemen, another member of the panel was the physician Joseph-Ignace Guillotin, now best remembered for the decapitation device he advocated, which later was used on both Bailly and Lavoisier. The fourth member of the panel was the American ambassador to France, Benjamin Franklin. The principal issue to be resolved by these men was the question of whether or not Mesmer had discovered a new physical fluid.

The commission observed blindfolded patients who were sitting in front of powerful magnets and asked the patients to describe their sensations. The commission compared their responses to those made when fake magnets were substituted without the subjects' knowledge. As you might imagine from the simplistic test, the results didn't favor Mesmer. Some subjects responded to the supposed magnetic effects even when the real magnets were not present.

The panel concluded that there was no evidence of a magnetic fluid and that magnetic healing was the result of the patient's belief in it and of the influence of imagination, suggestion, and imitation.[19] The panel's report opened by stating, "Animal magnetism might well exist without being useful, but it cannot be useful if it does not exist."[20]

Mesmer countered the findings by requesting that the panel select patients with various stubborn neuropsychiatric problems, and contrast the results of his treatment with those that the best conventional treatment could provide. The panel refused. Public sessions held before the Academy to discuss Mesmer's ideas reportedly "degenerated into chaos, and finally his thesis and system were rejected."[21] Understandably soured on Paris, Mesmer returned to Germany, where he died at age 81, the controversy his ideas spawned by no means settled. In many respects, it continues to this day.

Further advances that have contributed dramatically to today's understanding of magnet therapy were made in the late 1700s by Luigi Galvani, a professor of medicine at the University of Bologna, and Alessandro Volta, a physicist at the University of Pavia. It was Galvani who first observed a frog's legs twitching when touched by iron. His conclusion, though partially mistaken, was that electricity was hidden in the nerves. Volta took Galvani's observation a step further and concluded that a previously unsuspected kind of electricity existed (at the time, only static electricity was known). His research led him to the invention of the battery.

From 1799 to 1804, the German naturalist and statesman Alexander von Humboldt took a scientific journey through South America, Cuba, and Mexico. Having taken measurements, Humboldt concluded that the earth's magnetic intensity was dependent on latitude. Following his explorations, he organized the first simultaneous observation of the geomagnetic field at various locations throughout the world.

Beginning in the early 1800s, Humboldt, along with the German physicist Wilhelm Weber, who devised an electromagnetic telegraph in 1833, and the German mathematician and astronomer Carl Friedrich Gauss, who proposed an absolute system of magnetic units, organized the Göttingen Magnetic Union. From 1836 to 1841, simultaneous observations of the earth's magnetic field were made in nonmagnetic huts at 50 locations throughout the world. This activity marked the beginning of the international magnetic observatory system. Shortly thereafter, in 1847, the photographic recorder, which could provide a truly continuous record of the earth's geomagnetic field, was introduced at the Greenwich Observatory near London.

MAGNETIC AMERICA

Meanwhile, in the 1800s in the United States, magnet therapy was rising in popularity, likely spurred, at least in part, by Benjamin Franklin's experiments with electricity, and, by the eternal desire for quick, painless cures and the readiness of serious medical practitioners and quacks alike to provide them.

Elisha Perkins, a Connecticut physician, received a 1796 patent for a "magnetic tractor" device a little over three inches long. When held in the hand of a therapist and repeatedly and gently stroked across the affected part of the patient's body toward the heart, the tiny device drew off the surcharge of "putrid" electric fluid that Perkins believed caused pain. Perkins sold the tractors for prices that ranged from $25 per pair to $8 per pair per thousand, in an act that one author calls an attempt to monopolize their use, quoting Perkins as saying he hoped they would make "me and mine as rich as we ought to wish to be." Jacques Quen believes, however, that Perkins's motivation for increasing his devices' distribution was more complex than merely financial.[22]

Perkins's inflated confidence in his invention led him, like so many before him, to exaggerate its effectiveness. He claimed it would cure not only inflammatory disorders, but also the plague and yellow fever, and would aid "in calming and sedating violent cases of insanity."[23] Alas, when Perkins contracted yellow fever in 1799, he treated himself unsuccessfully with his device, and died eight days after the onset of symptoms.

It was not until almost a half century later that *The History and Philosophy of Animal Magnetism* was written and published in Boston by a "Practical Magnetizer." Around the same time, Phineas Quimby, a follower of Mesmer, established a magnetic healing practice in Portland, Maine. One of his successes was a patient named Mary Patterson, later to become Mary Baker Eddy, founder of Christian Science. Originally a proponent of mesmerism, Eddy came to believe that prayer was the only source of healing and that animal magnetism was "malicious" and "the action of error in all its forms."[24]

The popularity of magnets as healing devices soared in the post–Civil War era. The Sears Roebuck catalog advertised a wide range of magnetic jewelry and apparel, presumably able to heal just about any ailment of the human body from head to toe, including menstrual cramps, impotence, and baldness. Magnetic boot soles could be purchased for 18 cents a pair. Popular magnetic salves and liniments were sold over the counter and peddled by traveling charismatic (magnetic?) medicine men. Toward the end of the century, Daniel Palmer, later to become famous as the founder of the Palmer method of chiropractic, opened Palmer's School of Magnetic Cure in Davenport, Iowa, emphasizing massage and manipulation, as well as magnet therapy.[25]

During this time, the undisputed king of magnetic healers (some would say hucksters) was Dr. C. J. Thacher of Chicago, founder of the Magnetic Company. Thacher's company pamphlet promised "a plain road to health without the use of medicine." According to Thacher, it was the magnetic force of the sun, conducted through the iron content of the blood, that was responsible for life, and health. Disease occurred when stressful lifestyles and environmental factors interfered with the flow of that force. "Magnetism properly applied will cure every curable disease no matter what the cause," he wrote in his mail order advertising.

Thacher's company advocated magnetic clothing as the most efficient means to expedite cures, and provided almost every kind of garment for the human body — another head-to-toe cure-all. A complete costume, containing 700 magnets, offered the hope of "full and complete protection of all the vital organs of the body."

For an interview with a reporter, Thacher was well dressed in a stylish costume of "magnetic cap, a magnetic waistcoat, magnetic stocking liners, and magnetic insoles." He explained his motive as one of spreading the light to rescue humanity.

"I can cure anything," he boasted. "I will compel the authorities to take notice of my methods." Thacher suggested that "authorities" provide him with 10 ailing persons on whom he could place his magnetic shields, thereby restoring the "harmonious vibrations of the brain" so they would be well. "Paralysis? An easy problem. Had five cases . . . Cured 'em right off. Winked. Spoke. Got up and walked. Paralysis? Pish!"[26]

Unfortunately, one or two sensational shams can easily obscure, trivialize, and create unwarranted suspicion about the work of hundreds of legitimate physicians and researchers. And "the authorities" have historically been all too willing to throw the baby out with the bathwater in an attempt to protect the public interest.

THE ELECTRIC AGE JOLTS MAGNET THERAPY

When the German physicist Heinrich Hertz generated electromagnetic waves at radio frequencies in 1888, and the Serbian-American inventor Nikola Tesla lit up the Chicago World's Fair in 1893 with the first AC power system, the stage was set for medical breakthroughs. By the turn of the century, medical schools viewed electrotherapy as a legitimate area of study, much like the ever-growing field of radiology, and medical textbooks devoted chapters to the use of magnetism and electricity for treating a host of neurological and emotional disorders.

In an echo of Mesmer, doctors once again began to utilize electromagnetic therapy to relieve all types of pain, as well as to treat emotional disorders, arthritis, sleep disorders, and headaches. As you might expect, with the dissemination of all sorts of bogus theories and contraptions, each associated with lavish claims, people became disenchanted with magnetism as a cure. Further, following World War II, chemical-based medical advances such as antibiotics and cortisone provided remedies that were more easily predictable, repeatable, and quantifiable. Magnet therapy lost its allure — until, that is . . .

THE BIZARRE CASE OF DR. REICH

Practically everyone agrees that Wilhelm Reich was brilliant. Some say he went crazy; others say he was a clairvoyant who was killed for delivering a message that angered the government. Whatever the truth, his story has certainly added to the present-day controversy over electromagnetism.

Reich, an Austrian psychoanalyst and student of Sigmund Freud who emigrated to the United States in 1939, researched the effects on humans of such environmental pollutants as electromagnetism and radioactivity. He also became enamored of a substance he called "orgone energy," which, he asserted, functioned as a form of life energy. In connection with his study of orgone, he developed a contraption called the orgone energy accumulator, a device that he believed could attract and store up orgone. He believed that by sitting in the box, a person could recharge his or her energy.

Like Mesmer, and other "healers" before him, Reich attracted an enthusiastic following. He was one of the first to make claims about environmental pollution, particularly pollution associated with nuclear explosions, and that such pollution was starting to affect orgone activities adversely. In a conspiracy-lover's move in the early 1950s, the Food and Drug Administration issued an injunction ordering Reich to stop promoting the orgone energy accumulator. Ignoring the injunction, he was sentenced to a federal penitentiary, where he died in 1957. Some ardent supporters feel that he died a political prisoner.

Was Reich merely a man whose ideas were ahead of his time? Perhaps. Certainly his ideas were a precursor to present-day concerns about the effects of environmental pollutants and the influence of electromagnetic fields on the human body. We now know, thanks to the development of sophisticated scientific devices and studies associated with them, that electromagnetic fields can, in fact, have biological effects.

MAGNETS TODAY

As we will show in the next chapter, researchers have achieved remarkable positive results using weak electromagnets or permanent magnets of various strengths to speed up the healing of wounds and bone fractures, and to treat anxiety, depression, insomnia, and even certain cancers. For pain sufferers, the good news includes inducing anesthesia and reducing or eliminating a wide range of chronic pain.

Today, magnet therapy has been officially accepted as a medical procedure in Germany, Japan, Israel, Russia, and 45 other countries for the treatment of arthritis, back pain, bursitis, carpal tunnel syndrome, headaches, sinus headaches, tennis elbow, and many other inflammatory, orthopedic, and neurological problems.

Magnetism is a force as old and fundamental as the earth itself. Moreover, its beneficial medical effects have been intimated for probably as long as man has been alive. We can easily imagine some prehistoric medicine man slapping a lodestone to the aching back of his chief hunter and then basking in the gratitude of his patient — and of the tribe as a whole — when the "magical" cure worked.

But of course, neither that putative cave-dwelling medicine man nor the centuries of healers who followed him knew how magnets worked or why. As magic was systematically debunked, magnet therapy fell into disrepute. Now modern medicine has come full circle. We have moved, as Robert O. Becker puts it, from the shaman-healer's mysterious energies to a scientific understanding of the body's life energies. "What is emerging is a new paradigm of life, energy and medicine."[27]

Chapter Three

MAGNETS WORK

A chemistry teacher asked his class to tell him the chief property of water.

"It quenches thirst," one student said. "It dissolves substances"; "It prompts life," others offered. As the teacher shook his head, they went further afield: "It ionizes salts"; "It turns anhydrous copper sulphate blue."

"No, no!" he thundered at them. "The chief property of water is that it is *wet!*"

Sometimes the most obvious facts are the hardest to recognize — and they are often the hardest to prove. We all know beyond a shadow of doubt that we would fall to our death if we were to jump off the Empire State Building, but, short of actually doing so, can we *prove* it? Probably, but not too easily.

So it is with the use of magnets to reduce or eliminate pain. It's true, they work. People have been demonstrating that to themselves for centuries. Is it provable?

Brenda Adderly, this book's coauthor, suffered from chronic back pain for about six months while she was writing her previous book (probably as a result of sitting glued to her word processor for many hours a day). As soon as she started working on this book, the pain returned, even worse. Naturally, given the book's subject, she immediately strapped a magnet to her back. Within a few hours the pain lessened. Within three days, it disappeared, and, now, even without wearing the magnets, no matter how many hours she sits before her word processor, she is pain-free. Proof that magnets work, surely.

No, not really. For what Brenda may be experiencing, while certainly of great comfort to her, may be from the placebo effect of the magnet. Because she believes that the magnet works, her brain may be telling her that she has no pain, and may simply be refusing to feel it. Mesmer revisited!

Of course, common sense suggests that some 40 million Japanese could not all be consistently fooled into believing that magnets really work and that aspirin and other analgesics (to which, of course, they have just as easy access as Americans do) are often not needed. Common sense notwithstanding, even with large numbers of people experiencing the same benefits the placebo effect remains a theoretically possible explanation.

To *prove* that permanent magnets can relieve pain, we have to resort to carefully controlled studies of comparable groups of people, some of whom alleviated their pain through the use of magnets, while others, using pieces of metal they *thought* were magnetized, showed significantly *less* pain reduction.

Clearly, that's a tall order. Magnet therapy only occasionally yields instant results. It usually takes a few days of constant use, and the difference between a magnetized and an unmagnetized piece of metal is easy enough to detect (especially if more than a single magnet is involved). For example, people asked to wear a necklace of several magnets strung together would be likely to recognize pretty quickly if they weren't magnetized. Therefore, conducting a true placebo-controlled study is exceedingly difficult.

An alternative approach to proving that magnet therapy works would be to place two pieces of metal, one magnetized, the other not, on opposite, equally painful, parts of the body — for example, two arthritic hands. Here again two obvious problems arise. One is that pain is rarely identical between any two areas of the body. The other is that unless the effect of the magnets is very rapid, the sufferer is again likely to divine which of the two pieces of metal is the magnetized one.

A third way of conducting a placebo-controlled test on humans is to use real magnets and unmagnetized metal pieces alternately on the same individuals to see whether there are differences in result. Here again, the likelihood of the users discovering which piece of metal is a magnet and which one isn't is high, and any results from such a test are therefore questionable.

Finally, there is the possibility of animal experiments. There the placebo effect obviously does not play a role, but another problem arises. How do you get feedback from animals about the degree of pain reduction?

Given these problems in obtaining accurate measurements of permanent magnets' effect on pain, it is hardly surprising that not many studies with unarguably rigorous protocols have been conducted. Nevertheless, as this chapter will recount, sufficient evidence exists to convince most of us that magnet therapy works. Then again, there are always some unregenerate cynics who doubt everything until no room for doubt is left. They are the overskeptical critics who laughed at the absurdity of the Wright Brothers' ambition, and "proved" Pasteur's ideas about bacteria to be totally absurd.

THE STATE OF THE RESEARCH

Before we proceed to the evidence supporting our contention about the efficacy of *static magnetism* (permanent magnets) in pain reduction, allow us to digress to discuss what importance, if any, the copious research on *electromagnetism* may have.

Far more research has been done in this area for three main reasons. The first is that since, by its nature, electromagnetic therapy is likely to be conducted in a hospital, clinic, or laboratory, it is easily controlled by the researcher. The second is that because the duration of each treatment is short (although treatments may be repeated daily, and extend over lengthy time spans) and because patients do not feel the pulsing magnetism (except, of course, to the extent that it improves their condition), test and control groups can easily be kept ignorant of whether they are actually receiving an electromagnetic treatment or not. For the control group, the researcher simply does not switch on the machine. Consequently, test and control groups can be accurately compared and the placebo effect fairly easily accounted for.

Finally, since electromagnetism is frequently used to cure objectively quantifiable conditions — as distinct from alleviating pain, which is largely subjective — the results can be more easily measured. The time a bone takes to knit is less likely to be affected by the sufferer's hope that the treatment will work. Moreover, when this experiment is conducted on an animal and it is proved that electromagnetic force causes a horse's bones to knit substantially faster than they do under otherwise identical conditions, the case is closed to further debate.

Thus an extremely important question is whether and to

what extent research on electromagnetic treatments is relevant to treatments with permanent magnets. To summarize our thinking: The research findings on the effects of electromagnetism, while not fully translating to static magnetism, offer strong circumstantial evidence supporting the efficacy of permanent magnets in treating pain. When coupled with the direct studies on permanent magnetism, the evidence is quite compelling indeed. In this judgment, we are joined by many others: Dr. Ronald Lawrence, for example.

Lawrence is a clinical professor of medicine at UCLA, a graduate of the British Institute of Homeopathy, and a trained acupuncturist, who studied this ancient healing art in China. He has had a long and distinguished career in pain medicine. Many years ago, with John Bonita, he founded the Association for the Study of Pain. Later, at the University of Washington, he operated the first pain clinic in the world.

Lawrence virtually invented osteopuncture (acupuncture of the bones) and in the 1980s was invited by the Chinese government to advise them on the treatment of pain. He was closely involved with the development of magnets for curing the ailments of horses, and thereby helped Fabio Nor of Norfields build a prosperous business in the United States selling magnets to racehorse stables.

After more than a decade, Dr. Lawrence continues to be a spokesman on all matters related to alternative medicine for the Los Angeles County Medical Association. Until his mid-sixties, he remained a competitive marathon runner, and "for variety" he was the official physician attached to a successful ascent of Mount Everest. His remarkable life, coupled with his knowledge, experience, and achievements in both traditional and alternative medicine, make him an authority worth listening to.

THE PAIN RELIEF BREAKTHROUGH

"I have found an 85 percent effective rate [of pain relief] using permanent magnets," Lawrence explained. "Higher than anything you could expect, better than most medicines."

Then he went on to detail why, in his view, they work to some extent in the same way as electromagnets. "I used to think that the mechanisms were very different. Now, I'm coming to the realization — and some research is showing — that stationary or permanent magnets do their work by creating pulsed fields *because of their wearer's movement.* . . . You roll around in bed. You get up and walk. You are creating a moving magnetic field since your body is moving.

"Faraday was the one who showed us that moving a piece of metal inside a magnetic field creates an electric current in the metal. And a nerve is analogous to a wire. So I'm trying to measure currents generated in the finger by putting a magnet on the wrist."

Dr. W. Ross Adey, former distinguished professor of medicine (neurology) at the Loma Linda University School of Medicine in Loma Linda, California, subscribes to a similar view. He reaches a conclusion similar to Lawrence's when he says, "From Faraday's historic research, electromagnetic fields arise from *moving electric charges.* Thus, any tissue interaction with permanent magnetic fields can only occur with moving electric charges — ions, moving cells in blood, or movement of the whole body through permanent magnetic fields."[1]

If Lawrence's theory is correct, there would be significant similarities between permanent and electromagnetism. Those similarities would explain why so many people (and animals) appear to benefit from permanent magnets as much or almost as much as they do from electromagnets.

Nevertheless, there are also differences between pulsing electromagnetism and permanent magnetism, and no reader should fall into the trap of believing that the impressive positive findings about the efficacy of pulsing electromagnetism alone *necessarily* prove the efficacy of permanent magnets. The *proof* that permanent magnets work — and that the endless testimonies to their efficacy are more than misobservations based on the placebo effect — must rest on the more limited research conducted on permanent magnets themselves.

HOW ELECTROMAGNETISM AND
PERMANENT MAGNETISM DIFFER

Pulsing electromagnetism and permanent magnetism differ in two respects. One is that electromagnetism can be considerably more powerful. As we discussed in chapter 1, far higher gauss levels can be achieved in electromagnets than in permanent ones. This hardly matters in practice, however, since numerous studies of electromagnetic therapy (and this applies to nearly all the research we will discuss) used magnetism no stronger than what is achievable with permanent magnets.

Moreover, there's ample research on, and a powerful theoretical argument in favor of, using only very low levels of magnetism for therapeutic purposes. The theory is that although the scientific community has not yet broken the code to understand exactly how or why magnetism works therapeutically, nearly everyone agrees (as we will discuss in chapter 5) that part of its effectiveness involves interaction with the body's own magnetic energy. But the level of the body's electrical impulses and, therefore, of the magnetic fields they generate, while vital, is exceedingly low. There would, therefore, seem to be no great need or advantage in using high levels of outside magnetism to influence low levels of internal magnetism. Killing a fly with a rolled-up newspaper leaves it just as dead as attacking it with a sledgehammer, and the greater dexterity the newspaper permits makes it far more likely that you'll hit the fly in the first place.

The second difference between the two types of magnetism is the pulsing nature of electromagnetism. Even though many of the most impressive results from electromagnetic therapy have been achieved with very low frequencies (as little as 2 Hz [hertz], or two pulses per second), the fact remains that pulsed magnetism is as different from permanent magnetism as, by analogy, a massaging shower head is different from a straight shower, or a massage where pressure is applied with a vibrating instrument is different from one with the same pressure applied without vibration. As Dr. Riva Sanseverino of the Instituto di Fisiologica Umana (the Institute of Human Physiology) at the University of Bologna and his colleagues point out in their 11-year study of 3,014 patients, "interrupted stimulations are *more* [emphasis ours] effective than the continuous ones since sensitive receptors and excitable membranes are usually stimulated by energy variations."[2]

It is easy to agree with these researchers, especially since the size and scope of their study is so impressive. Clearly they are not suggesting that uninterrupted stimulation has no effect; merely that energy variations make treatment *more* effective. We have no reason to doubt that, but such treatments, while more effective, are also impractical for many patients. Permanent magnets, while perhaps less effective per treatment, have the advantage of being readily available to all patients all the time.

THE CASE FOR ELECTROMAGNETISM

Since we've mentioned the definitive study by Sanseverino, let us continue our discussion about electromagnetism by describing that research in more detail, as a foundation for our discussion about permanent magnets.

This study, published in 1992 in *Panminerva Med,* an established Italian medical journal, looked at the effects of pulsed magnetic fields (MF) on chronic and acute conditions existing in diseases of different joints, with the presence of phlogistic process (*phlogistic,* literally "flaming," means an inflamed area or an inflammation, and implies a very painful condition). The researchers state, "Optimal parameters for MF applications were sought and then applied for 11 years."

Pulsed magnetic fields of extremely low frequencies and intensities were administered to 3,014 patients. The resulting pain relief, recovery of joint mobility, and maintenance of improved conditions were rated "good" or "poor." The researchers conducted careful statistical analyses on their findings to make sure that "the results were not casual."

The results were certainly not that. They were overwhelming. There was an average of 78.8 percent "good" results, 21.2 percent "poor" results. Moreover, the criteria by which a result was found to be "good" were tough. Some mild improvement was not sufficient. Rather, "good" meant at least (1) the disappearance of pain in the affected region; (2) a 40 to 50 percent increase in joint mobility following one treatment, rising to 50 to 100 percent with repeated treatments; and (3) the maintenance of the benefit achieved by each treatment.

Clearly, the quality of these results speaks for itself. But the researchers were very careful in two other respects and thereby further improved the value of their findings:

The first had to do with safety and side effects, which they studied quite closely (and which we will cover in the next chapter).

They concluded that there simply was not a problem. "Negative results and undesired side effects have never been observed," they stated flatly.

Of course, this entire story could still conceivably be written off as the result of the placebo effect. Here, too, the researchers were careful. During the course of this longitudinal probe, they conducted a double-blind study (that is, neither the patients nor the investigators knew which subjects were getting the real treatment and which were getting the decoy or placebo treatment) to prove that the results were physically based and not psychogenic. To this end, some patients were chosen to be subjected to the same procedure as other patients but the MF generator was kept turned off. Neither the patient nor the physiotherapist was aware of the control. "Since all 142 patients already had previous MF experience," the researchers write, "they were surprised at the absolute absence of any benefit from the control therapy." One week after the false MF experience, they received a regular MF treatment, most obtaining about the same result as they had in the past. Subsequently, they were told about the control therapy.

Given the length and size of the overall study, and the elimination of any reasonable possibility that the results came from a placebo effect, it is not surprising that the researchers concluded that due to the high percentage of good results and the absence of both negative results and undesired side effects, magnetic field treatment is an excellent physical therapy for joint diseases.

NECK PAIN STUDY

A much smaller, more traditional, and specific double-blind study was conducted at Mater Misericordiae Hospital in Dublin, Ireland. There researchers studied 20 patients with neck pain that had persisted for at least eight weeks. For the first three weeks of the study, 10 patients were exposed to a low-energy but high-frequency electromagnetic field. The other 10 patients (the placebo group) were subjected to the same procedures, but without any magnetic force being applied. At the end of the three-week period, 9 of the patients who were actually treated reported "moderately" or "much" less pain. Their range of movement increased correspondingly. Only 2 of the patients in the placebo group reported any improvement.

During the next three weeks, all 20 patients wore electromagnetic collars. At the end of that time, 17 of the 20 were at least "moderately" improved, leaving the researchers to conclude that this sort of electromagnetic treatment is "frequently successful and without side effects."[3]

PARKINSON'S DISEASE CASE STUDY

A very different but, in its own way, equally persuasive study was conducted by Dr. Reuven Sandyk and his associates at the Democrition University of Thrace in Greece. This study, the case history of a single individual, was published in the prestigious, peer-reviewed *International Journal of Neuroscience* in 1992. It dealt with the effects of very weak electromagnetic fields on the dyskinesia (uncontrollable movements) that is often a side effect of the drug levodopa in Parkinson's patients. As Sandyk (who, incidentally, has conducted a slew of research on a variety of magnetic therapies) explains, "Despite its efficacy [in managing Parkinson's], chronic levodopa therapy is associated with the development of several complications, including psychiatric symptoms and involuntary movement disorders, both of which limit its long-term usefulness."[4]

The researchers describe in graphic detail the drug side effects suffered by their 62-year-old patient, who was diagnosed with

Parkinson's in 1980 and was able to control the disease for 8 years by taking levodopa. Aside from the Parkinson's, the patient was healthy in all other respects until the dyskinetic symptoms appeared. And they were quite unpleasant. Within 30 to 45 minutes after taking a dose of levodopa, the man experienced severe dyskinesias and dystonic movements (twitching, writhing, flexing, and spastic motions) of the face, neck, extremities, and trunk. They lasted up to two hours, severely restricting his daily activities and limiting his ability to care for himself. Every morning the patient experienced painful tonic extension of his right foot and an almost continuous dull ache over his left shoulder and lower back muscles. The researchers reported that the patient "appeared to be distressed and anxious." Hardly surprising!

To deal with the problem, the researchers applied an extremely weak electromagnetic pulse to the patient's head for only six minutes. The frequency of the stimulation was twice a second (2 Hz), and the intensity of the magnetic field a tiny 7.5 picotesla (a picotesla is one-trillionth of a tesla; 1 tesla = 10,000 gauss). Within one day, the results were spectacular. The man was able to rapidly rise from his chair without assistance. His gait became almost normal, and few rapid, jerky, involuntary movements followed his ingestion of levodopa. The patient reported that he no longer experienced stiffness or difficulty turning in bed; the painful dystonic postures of the right foot no longer occurred; and the aches in the shoulder and back muscles had disappeared. To top it off, the patient reported a marked improvement in both his relaxation and his sexual arousability!

Obviously, in a case-history study there can be no control, and the vaunted placebo effect could account for all the improvement; however, in this sort of extreme case that seems unlikely. The side effects the patient suffered are well known to occur some time after levodopa treatment is started, but their onset after eight years is far more likely to be physically based than psychosomatic. The benefit of the electromagnetic pulse treatment lasted about 72 hours, after which time the drug side effects reappeared but could be eliminated again by a further application of the electromagnetic therapy. We share the conviction of the researchers that this man's case demonstrates the "potentially powerful effects of weak magnetic fields in the treatment of Parkinsonism and associated complications of levodopa therapy," even though "[the electromagnetism] mode of action in Parkinsonism remains elusive."

MULTIPLE SCLEROSIS STUDY

Dr. Reuven Sandyk, now associated with Tuoro College in Dix Hills, New York, conducted an equally interesting case study, this one on the effect of an extremely low electromagnetic field on a 55-year-old woman with multiple sclerosis (MS).[5] MS is a devastating disease that gradually destroys the ability to walk, breathe freely, sit comfortably, maintain bladder control, see, and eventually, to think clearly.

When the patient came to Sandyk, she was in bad shape. Her legs were numb. She could not stand without a cane, and she could hardly walk at all. She was incontinent and her speech was garbled and hoarse. She felt exhausted, had memory lapses, and found it difficult to do simple arithmetic. Her vision had faded to the point where she could only barely read a newspaper. She was hardly able to draw even a very simple picture of a house.

This woman was exposed to electromagnetic treatments. The first treatment, which lasted 20 minutes, was a sham; the magnet device was simply not turned on. The second treatment, lasting the same length of time, exposed her to an electromagnetic force of 7.5 picotesla with a frequency of 5 Hz.

The results, even as couched in Dr. Sandyk's conservative, muted words, were spectacular: "While placebo magnetic treatment produced no change in the patient's motor disability or drawing performance, treatment with MF resulted in an almost immediate clinical response, with the patient reporting improvement of vision with images appearing clearer and brighter." She rose from her chair faster, was less unsteady, and even walked for several minutes without the support of a walker. She reported that she had immediately experienced a feeling of relaxation and mood elevation, and it was noted that she smiled spontaneously several times.

The woman was asked to repeat the drawing of a house and showed improved performance, adding further details that suggested enhancement of "visuoconstructive abilities." A week after the electromagnetic treatment, the woman reported that she had felt more energetic and more optimistic during the preceding week. She said her head felt "clearer," and her concentration had improved. Sleep had also improved, in part due to "stabilization of her bladder functions."

Her legs felt stronger, the numbness in the lower extremities was less, and her balance was better. She was able to walk in her apartment with greater stability, sometimes using only a cane. Best of all, she reported no side effects.

Again, this is a case study of only a single patient and, as Sandyk states, "clearly further studies involving a larger cohort of patients are required." For now, the study adds yet another impressive plank of evidence for the growing edifice of proof that electromagnetic therapy works.

DEPRESSION STUDY

Another set of scientists, led by Dr. Mark George and affiliated with the National Institutes of Health, have been looking at the effect of electromagnetic therapy on severe depression. In 1995, they reported some of their findings.[6] Choosing six medication-resistant people (with a mean age of 46.5 years) on whom no other treatment was having much impact, they administered a rapidly repeated electromagnetic stimulus each morning for a week. The overall results were pleasing. While two patients showed no response, two did show a slight but "meaningful" improvement. As the researchers describe it, clearly suppressing their delight only with difficulty, the remaining two "had a robust clinical antidepressant response."

The researchers found that the only meaningful side effect was a mild headache that disappeared with the use of ordinary analgesics. They concluded that their pilot studies demonstrate that the use of electromagnetic therapy is a safe and, most probably, broadly effective procedure. Continuing in their work with new double-blind studies under way, they report "encouraging" results with the first few test subjects.

A FEW OTHER STUDIES

Some studies of the effect of electromagnetism are so dramatic that even in the absence of any placebo controls, the results cannot be ignored. In this category is a whole body of Russian research, much of which has not been translated into English. One such study is typical of many.

In 1982, V. V. Kuz'menko and Y. D. Katz studied 240 amputees who had limb stumps and what the researchers describe as "painful syndromes." The pain was treated with a home apparatus that emitted a weak magnetic field. The results: 94 percent showed some reduction in pain, and two-thirds of those reported that the pain had almost completely disappeared.[7] While we have no doubt that the placebo effect played a significant role, it seems exceedingly unlikely that it could fully account for anything close to this success rate. In fact, in a carefully conducted study of placebo effects in electromagnetic therapy, a team of researchers at Johns Hopkins found that only 10 to 16 percent of patients "will consistently respond to treatments that have no possibility of being directly therapeutic."[8]

Throughout the world, pulsed electromagnetic fields have been authoritatively reported to effect cures or to greatly reduce medical problems — and so to alleviate or eliminate pain associated with them — not only in the examples we have given here, but in accelerated bone repair, nerve regeneration, skin ulcer healing, recovery from damage to soft tissues, and tendinitis.[9]

"Bioelectrical Applications in Medicine," an article written by six distinguished researchers in 1992, cites an astonishing body of evidence demonstrating that electromagnetism is effective in bone and cartilage repair, soft-tissue and wound healing, neural tissue growth and regeneration, behavioral problems, "acupuncture-style" pain reduction, modifications in the pineal gland's production of melatonin, immune system effects, arthritis treatment, and cellular and subcellular effects on tumors.[10]

That's quite a list.

However, the researchers state that, as of the date of their publication, there were no known published journal articles that demonstrated, via clinical trials, the effectiveness of *permanent* magnets. While that statement may have been less than fully informed even back then, it is even less true today. There is now quite a lot of evidence about the efficacy of permanent magnetic fields.

THE CASE FOR PERMANENT MAGNETIC FIELDS

One exceedingly important medical use of electromagnetism is with the destruction of certain cancer cells. Since our topic is pain relief, we do not intend to probe into this area in too much depth, but we want to touch on it for two reasons. The first is that in the field of cancer cell destruction, we have the best example of electromagnetism and permanent magnetism both having a similar beneficial effect. Of course, this does not mean that the two forces work in the same way or with the same degree of efficacy. It does, however, provide another hint that the dramatic effects of electromagnetic therapy, as proved by copious research (only a small portion of which we have summarized here), may to some extent be shared by permanent magnetic therapy. Our second reason for touching on this subject is that it shows yet again how very powerful a tool magnetic therapy can be. As far back as 1961, Indumati Mulay and L. N. Mulay of the University of Cincinnati reported in the prestigious British journal *Nature* that they had conducted a controlled experiment involving a permanent magnet and mouse tumor cells. Slides of tumor cells placed between the poles of a magnet with a strength about 4,000 gauss showed "complete degeneration" after 18 hours; identical cells not exposed to the magnetism showed normal growth. The researchers repeated the experiment several times with the same results.[11]

In 1963, Madeleine F. Barnothy, associate professor of pharmacy at the University of Illinois, described a series of experiments that she and her husband had conducted on mice to determine the effects of fixed magnetism on cancer. Barnothy wrote that her husband believed a magnetic field might be able to isolate the malignant tissues and perhaps induce a rejection or destruction of carcinoma.

He proved his point, she says. First, he inoculated 22 mice with cancer cells and, five days later, placed 6 of them in a permanent magnetic field. The rest were placed between identical dummy magnets (presumably to eliminate any possibility of someone suggesting that environmental factors played a role). The results? All of the controls died in the usual 14 to 20 days specific to the type of cancer being studied. Five of the treated mice rejected the already well-developed tumor in 20 to 30 days, and 4 of them were eventually completely healed.

Later, the Barnothys repeated their experiments at St. Francis Hospital in Evanston, Illinois, and found that while the mice exposed to the magnetic field did not reject the carcinoma and eventually all died, they lived 44 percent longer than the untreated mice, itself a signal achievement.[12]

Magnet experiments have been conducted since by many cancer researchers. For example, in 1994 D. B. Tata and colleagues at the University of Vermont reported to the American Association of Cancer Researchers' annual meeting that they had tested the effect of a strong permanent magnetic field (11.6 tesla) on mouse sarcoma, mouse leukemia, human breast carcinoma, human ovarian carcinoma, and human carcinoma of the mouth. The results were compared to those from control groups treated in exactly the same way but using magnet decoys.

The results were impressive. Compared to the controls, only the following levels of cancer cells in the experimental subjects survived:

Mouse sarcoma	4%
Mouse leukemia	10%
Human ovarian carcinoma	25%
Human carcinoma of the mouth	40%

Only human breast carcinoma appeared largely unaffected, with 92 percent as many cells surviving in the test subjects as in the control subjects.[13] Even with this exception, the results are cause for optimism.

An exceedingly important study on cancer cells largely confirming Tata's work was completed in 1996 by Dr. Raymond Raylman and his associates at the University of Michigan. Raylman reported in a paper published in *Bioelectromagnetics* that when three human tumor cell lines were exposed to a very strong permanent magnetic field for an extended period, the growth rate of magnet-exposed cells was lower than that for control groups. Furthermore, after several days of recovery, the cells regained the ability to reproduce at their normal rate without any consistent change in the normal cell cycle. Unfortunately, as the authors conclude, the mechanism for this behavior is as yet unknown."[14]

A recent case study suggests a static magnetic field emanating from a permanent magnet may also accelerate and stimulate bone grafting. This was the conclusion reached following the study of a surgically repaired hand injured by a gunshot. In that case study, on the fifth postoperative day, a permanent magnet was placed over the region of the patient's thumb where a bone graft had been set. The magnet was left there for the entire period of treatment. Within 5½ weeks, the thumb was stable, whereas the normal time period for such fusion is approximately 2 months. The accelerated healing was attributed to the magnetic field.[15] Here we have an application of a static magnetic field that heretofore had only been proved only with an electromagnetic field.

A different example of how the results of permanent magnets are often comparable to the results achieved by other proven — but more difficult to apply — treatments is a study conducted at Showa

University in Tokyo, Japan, comparing the effects of acupuncture and a permanent magnet on a pained muscle. The result of the study, which is discussed in a different context in chapter 5, was simple: The magnet proved to be just as effective at reducing pain as the acupuncture.[16]

PERMANENT MAGNETS AND IMMEDIATE PAIN

A formal study of the effect of permanent magnets in inhibiting immediate pain was conducted by Jack P. Prince, DDS, and published in the *American Journal of Acupuncture* in 1983. Dr. Prince found that when he did certain kinds of dental surgery, he needed to place four to six injections of a numbing agent into the tissue of the hard palate. These injections are among the most painful in dentistry. To ease his patients' discomfort, he decided to place permanent magnets on the upper and lower jaw before giving the injections. After many comparisons of working on both sides of the mouth during the same appointment and using the magnet on one side only, Prince has observed that there is definitely less discomfort on the side where the magnet is used. The patients most often reported that "the pain is less sharp on the side with the magnet."[17]

Of course, this finding should not be taken to mean that permanent magnets can immediately inhibit pain under all conditions. For example, a study conducted in 1977 by two researchers at the University of Manitoba in Canada found that just because you are wearing a magnetic bracelet does not mean you have a higher threshold of pain when you are exposed to increasing levels of radiant heat.[18] We have no idea whether a similar study has ever been conducted on, say, aspirin. We would not be surprised if two aspirins, which certainly tend to calm our mild headaches, nevertheless failed to make us more resistant to the pain of being burned!

WHIPLASH AND HEAD INJURY STUDIES

One of the most persuasive sets of studies showing that permanent magnetism can be highly effective in treating pain was reported by Dr. J. B. Baron, of the Centre Hospitalier Sainte-Anne of Paris, in 1983. The two studies he described were conducted respectively among 30 male volunteer firemen (a healthy bunch) between the ages of 20 and 30 and 700 patients suffering from painful whiplash or head injuries. Their purpose was to see whether the tendency to vertigo (either artificially induced in the healthy men or accident-produced in the injured population) could be corrected by permanent magnets. The short answer, drawn from an unfortunately very confused report, seems to be that indeed, it could. The researchers went on to say that magnets were so effective, they believed it would be appropriate to use them to prevent or cure vertigo and air sickness in astronauts.[19]

MENSTRUAL PAIN STUDY

Another type of pain on which permanent magnets have been tested and proved efficacious is dysmenorrhea, painful menstrual periods. Two Korean physicians at Seoul University outfitted 11 student nurses suffering from severe menstrual pain with permanent magnets of 800–1,200 gauss, and a second group of 12 nurses, also dysmenorrheic, with identical, but unmagnetized, pieces of metal. The magnets (and nonmagnets) were attached over the pubic bone and pain assessments on both groups were made after three hours, and again three hours after removing the magnets. The fact that the magnets were attached in the hospital and in a relatively inaccessible location on the body meant that the nurses could not easily determine which pieces of metal were magnets and which were the placebos. Both during use and after removal, the women treated with the real magnets experienced significantly more pain reduction than those wearing the nonmagnets.[20]

URETHRAL STENOSIS STUDY

Yet another study, this one conducted in Moscow, showed that permanent magnets had a salutary effect on the very painful childhood condition called urethral stenosis, a blockage of the urethra (either from shrinkage or scarring) that makes urination difficult, painful, or, in some extreme cases, impossible. Before 1982, the standard treatment (assuming that a full-scale operation was not immediately required) was to tunnel out the urethra — obviously a miserable procedure. Unfortunately, in most cases this resolved the problem only temporarily. Often the urethra would eventually shrink back to its previous constricted diameter. In 1983, Dr. E. A. Stepanov and his colleagues investigated the effect of permanent magnets on the condition. They were unsuccessful where the stricture of the urethra was more than 1 centimeter; however, in four out of five patients with shorter strictures, the technique worked as well and lasted longer than ordinary tunneling.[21]

SOME ADDITIONAL STUDIES

Another persuasive example of the beneficial effects of permanent magnetism was reported by a team of Russian physicians led by E. Z. Rabinovich, who found that exposing healing skin to a magnetic field for 10 to 12 days improved the skin's ability to take in oxygen. Similarly, they reported, exposing skin grafts to a permanent magnetic field for 22 to 26 hours has the same effect. As a result of these improvements in the skin's "breathing" ability, the wounds healed faster, and there was naturally less pain.[22]

The positive effect of permanent magnets is also demonstrated by a 1996 Israeli study done on knee inflammation (synovitis) artificially induced in rats. Synovitis in humans is a very painful condition. This study showed that after exposure to a permanent magnet of 3,800 gauss, inflammation decreased dramatically. In the test rats, only 2 out of 10 knees showed continued inflammation; in the control group, 8 out of 10 knees remained seriously inflamed, and most of them showed symptoms resembling rheumatoid arthritis. The test group's inflammatory score was 3.4, the control group's 6.8, a very meaningful difference indeed. The researchers' conclusion is obvious: Continuous magnetic field treatment is an effective method of decreasing the inflammatory process of synovitis and "may serve as an adjuvant therapy for patients with inflammatory arthritis such as rheumatoid arthritis or psoriatic arthritis." They did add, correctly and conservatively, that controlled human studies are needed to evaluate the *clinical* relevance of such results.[23]

Let us conclude with an informal study conducted by Dr. Ronald Lawrence. He had 14 patients with carpal tunnel syndrome wear magnets on their painful wrists for a week. Then, rather than rely on their subjective judgment about pain reduction (which, without a control group, would have been hard to assess anyhow), he measured the conduction velocity of the nerves: that is, the speed with which electric impulses pass through the carpal tunnel in the wrist. In people who have the syndrome, the impulses are slowed by the pressure placed on the nerve. This was an entirely objective measurement; participants were not even told what Lawrence was planning to measure.

Lawrence reported: "Lo and behold, 12 of the 14 participants showed significant improvement. None got worse."

As we wrap up this partial review of the literature, keep in mind the image of Jim Colbert hitting golf balls vast distances; of Dr. Ron Lawrence's patients busily typing away, their carpal tunnel syndrome apparently cured; and of coauthor Brenda Adderly enjoying a pain-free back as she works on this and other books.

Perhaps all those otherwise sensible folks are merely experiencing placebo effects. Perhaps they have all been mesmerized or seduced by a 20th-century version of an alchemist's dream. But that's unlikely. In the foreground of our thought is the wealth of scientific data that support those personal observations. The jury has given its verdict loud and clear: Magnets can alleviate and sometimes eliminate pain.

Chapter Four

PERMANENT MAGNETS ARE SAFE

Are magnets safe? *"Absolutely,"* Dr. Ronald Lawrence assures us. "Magnetic resonance imaging (MRI) machines routinely expose patients to magnetic fields as high as 15,000 gauss with no negative effects." He goes on to explain, "Right this minute, if you took away the magnets in your environment, you and your whole house would fall apart."

MAGNETS ARE EVERYWHERE

In your refrigerator there are probably as many as 26 magnets. In your car, there are hundreds. Every electrical appliance has magnets in it. For instance, your air conditioner couldn't function without magnets. Nor could your heating system. Nor could your stereo or television.

"In fact," says Dr. Lawrence, "our whole planet would fall apart without its magnetic field of about half a gauss. . . ." If we lost that magnetic pull, we could not live on earth anymore. We'd be gone, and probably within less than a minute. As described so well in James Livingston's book *Driving Force: The Natural Magic of Magnets,* magnets really are a driving force.

Every study we quoted in chapter 3 confirms this view that

low levels of magnetic energy are entirely harmless. An experiment reported in *Aerospace Medicine* as long ago as 1961 indicated that exposure to an electromagnetic field of 8,800 to 14,000 gauss "did not significantly change the rate of young male animal growth, and did not significantly change the white blood count."[1]

An article in *Nature* three years later cited the use of permanent magnets with a strength of 5,000 gauss for extended periods on cultured cells with no negative side effects. No "gross lethal effects" were produced on mammalian cells either by powerful magnetic fields applied for short time periods or by lower field strengths that extended over many cell generations.[2]

On the other hand, some other researchers feel they have found some hints that permanent magnetism might cause some long-term damage. For example, a study reported in 1984 by a group of Italian researchers headed by G. Ardito of the University of Turin suggested that exposure of human lymphocyte cultures to a magnetic field of 740 gauss causes a slight increase in chromosome aberrations. While the sample of 10 males was small, there appeared to be a statistically significant difference that should not be ignored.[3]

Arthur Green, ScD, and Myron Halpern, PhD, conducted a similar experiment, testing hamster cells in magnetic fields from permanent horseshoe magnets at levels of 350 to 1,200 gauss. The results were unambiguous. No real significant difference in cell growth was found between cells grown in low magnetic fields and cells grown in the natural ambient field.

However, the experimenters, possibly concerned that their findings could mitigate against research that shows magnetism can inhibit the growth of *cancerous* cells, added an interesting caveat to their findings. They stated that their results do not disprove the thesis that magnetic fields of extremely low intensity (50 gamma) exert an effect on biological systems. "Close examination of the tissue culture data indicates a possible qualitative trend of effect even though a statistically significant quantitative difference is not demonstrated."[4]

THE SAFETY OF PERMANENT MAGNETS

Herein lies the problem, of course. How can the evidence that magnetism does something significant be so overwhelming, while most scientists insist that, at relatively low levels, magnetism is absolutely harmless?

The issue is, indeed, a complicated one. Our conclusion is that with permanent magnets, there is no health risk involved. Their level of magnetism is simply too low to do any harm. The body may *respond* to that level of magnetic force (as it may respond to low-level heat), but it cannot be harmed by it. If, and only if, the levels of electromagnetic pulsing become enormously higher than would occur from any normal exposure does even a reasonable possibility of harm start to exist.

Moreover, any possible harm that such high levels might cause in no way implies that low levels are also harmful. The appropriate analogy here is not a poison that is lethal in high doses and, while it may not kill you in lower quantities, is generally unlikely to do you any good. Rather, the correct analogy is heat (another form of energy), which is good, even essential, at low levels, a pleasure to feel when you warm your hands *in front of* a fire, but dangerous if you put your hands *into* the fire. A 1987 study commissioned by the World Health Organization indicated that in 40 years of research, the magnetic fields produced by permanent magnets have never been implicated in any mutagenic process.[5]

As we believe we proved in chapter 3, permanent and electromagnetism both have an important positive effect on the body, and particularly on pain. And the weight of research indicates that even at relatively high levels, and certainly at low ones, there is no convincing evidence that magnetism is harmful.

The reason both these statements can be true is that the general magnetic fields surrounding us are so dispersed and minor that we are simply unaffected by them, or, if affected at all, we recover almost instantly and show no adverse aftereffects. Were it otherwise, the human population would never have made it this far. Scientists believe that the earth's magnetism was once far higher than it is today. Natural events like thunderstorms cause surges of magnetic energy. Deposits of lodestone in Sweden, Norway, Romania, and Siberia, as well as in parts of New York State, Utah, and Minnesota, presumably have long exposed people living near them to magnetic fields whose strength is far above average. And none of these influences seem to have inhibited anyone's development. Clearly, our bodies are used to outside magnetic influences and can withstand them easily enough. If, as Becker maintains, we "swim" in a sea of energy, then we have evidently learned to do it well enough to avoid drowning!

And when that same magnetic energy is applied specifically to a painful area, it has been shown, over and over again, both in carefully controlled scientific experiments and in almost infinitely repeated personal experiences, that pain is reduced or eliminated.

Permanent magnets work. The question is, exactly *how* do they work? In the next chapter, we will provide what is known about that subject, and give our own ideas as to how permanent magnets relieve pain. The explanation will, to some degree, be speculative because no one fully understands all the aspects of how biomagnetism works.

A COUPLE OF SENSIBLE PRECAUTIONS

1. Before you use magnets or any other device, medication, or procedure, *always* check first with your doctor. Among other reasons for doing this, it may be quite undesirable to cure a persistent, *unexplained* pain before your doctor has observed it. That pain could be a symptom of something problematic that needs to be dealt with promptly. Check out what is causing the pain before you eliminate this symptom and thus make it harder to trace the underlying problem.

2. If you are pregnant, on any form of medication, or suffering from a chronic disease, do not use magnets (or any other device, medication, or procedure) without checking it out with the health care experts who are advising you on your condition. This is because anything new you do to your body may, in some way, interfere with or negate what you are already doing. (For example, it is obvious that you should not use magnet therapy if you are wearing a pacemaker that could be thrown off by a magnetic force.)

Beyond those self-evident but important caveats — warnings that apply to every medical product or procedure — we confidently agree with Dr. Lawrence: Permanent magnets are safe.

Chapter Five

HOW MAGNET THERAPY WORKS

The scientific community has detected many hints, and developed many theories, about how magnet therapy works, but it has not, as yet, come up with a complete, definitive, or universally accepted answer. The reason for this, we suspect, is that no single answer actually exists, because magnet therapy works through many different mechanisms. Thus there have to be several *layers* to the complicated answer to the simple question "How do magnets cure pain?"

For us, it is not the theories that are of primary importance, but the facts. And the fact is that permanent magnets do provide prompt and powerful pain relief for many patients. The research is equally clear that *electromagnetic* fields speed up the healing of bone fractures and soft-tissue injuries to a remarkable degree, and can be effective in treating stress-related disorders, including anxiety, insomnia, and depression, even in patients resistant to drugs. Unlike heat, X-rays, and other forms of energy, magnetic fields are not obstructed or reflected by bone or other impediments, and can reach structures deep in the body. More important, in contrast to some other nontraditional approaches permanent magnets are safe, relatively inexpensive, and essentially everlasting, making them extremely cost effective. These facts notwithstanding, we remain fascinated by the challenge of understanding the mechanism by which magnetism works.

We should add here that the fact that not everything is known about how magnetic energy works leaves room for practitioners to generate their own unlikely, and often extreme, theories. For example, one doctor maintains that "when negative magnetic energy is applied to a cell, the counterclockwise spin of the negatively charged cellular DNA pulls oxygen . . . into the cell." He goes on to explain that "all microorganisms (bacterial, viral, fungal) and parasites are positive magnetic energy driven and are, therefore, stunned or retarded by negative magnetic energy."[1] To date, such findings have in no way been substantiated.

IS IT INCREASED BLOOD FLOW?

The easiest part of the answer to the question "How do magnets work?"— the basal layer, so to speak — is the presumption that magnetic fields promote blood flow to the affected area. This effect has been shown clearly as it applies to *electromagnetism*. For example, in the Sanseverino research mentioned in chapter 3, the investigators observed vasodilation (increased blood flow through expanded blood vessels) after a single exposure to an electromagnetic field. This finding mirrored those of another study and was therefore of no surprise to the researchers.[2]

Of course, the fact that increased blood flow occurs under the impact of electromagnetic fields does not prove that it occurs in *permanent* magnetic fields. Many practitioners, however, are convinced that it does. Dr. Ronald Lawrence believes that as a result of permanent magnets being moved (as their wearers move), they generate microcurrents in the nerves near them that enhance blood flow. Lawrence reports that he has measured the blood flow in the finger after putting a magnet on the wrist and has found that within a minute there is a 300 percent increase in blood flow to the finger, *provided the wrist is moving.*

"What I do is measure blood flow in a patient's finger, then attach the magnet to the wrist and have the patient move the wrist very slightly — just 10 degrees up, 10 degrees back, 10 degrees to the right, 10 degrees back — and remeasure the flow," Lawrence says. He finds that without the wrist movement the blood flow does not increase, but with that movement people experience a palpable increase in blood flow. "When they touch their husband, or their boyfriend, or whoever, with one hand and then with the other, he can feel the difference in temperature," Lawrence says.

The fact that an increase in blood flow has curative and pain-reducing impact is, of course, well established. The blood carries away toxins, and brings in white blood cells (leukocytes), which work to reduce inflammation, reduce swelling, and speed a cure. All of this, of course, tends to decrease pain.

We have no doubt that this is one part of the reason magnets are effective. However, the speed of pain alleviation, the completeness of it, the fact that the system continues to work over long periods, and the observable fact that magnets clearly work far better than, say, a heating pad or Ben Gay ointment, both of which also bring blood to the surface, all strongly suggest that this is only one aspect of magnetism's efficacy and not a complete explanation. It may be only a small part of the full explanation at that.

DOES IT WORK LIKE ACUPUNCTURE?

One of the ideas many magnet practitioners are considering is the relationship between healing by permanent magnets and acupuncture points. Traditional acupuncture and its meridian systems (lines of energy), developed by the Chinese, has been practiced for more than 5,000 years.[3] Although one of the oldest known systems of healing, it was not until 1958 that acupuncture anesthesia for surgery was first used in China.[4] Introduction of the use of acupuncture analgesia in this country has had a major influence on pain research.[5]

The English word *acupuncture* comes from *acus,* "needle," and *pungere,* "to puncture or pierce." The Chinese word for acupuncture is *chen-chiou,* meaning "needle burn," which refers to the technique of moxibustion, in which the moxa herb (*Artemisia vulgaris*) is burned over a meridian point.[6]

Acupuncture involves inserting sterilized needles at specific acupuncture points along the 14 meridians and twirling them manually for stimulation, the theory being that imbalances in the meridian lines of the body would be expressed as pain and their stimulation via the needles would reduce the pain. Traditional theory does not refer to pain as much as it refers to restoring physical harmony along the meridians, with subsequent restoration of health.

Happily for those of us in pain today, we no longer need to rely on the sharp stone needles, called *pien,* used in bygone eras,[7] nor their replacement, needles made of bone or bamboo. Characteristic sensations described following the insertion of today's stainless steel needles into a point on the meridians include "tingling" and "numbness" or no feeling at all.

The research of Dr. Kim Bong Han of the University of Pyongyang in North Korea has led him to believe that the meridians, once thought to be invisible, are actually channels composed of a type of histological tissue hitherto undiscovered, which exist beneath the surface of the skin. According to Han, they have a thin membranous wall and are filled with a transparent, colorless fluid. A series of experiments by German scientists led to the conclusion that the meridians are pathways for electricity.[8]

Each meridian, with varying numbers of acupuncture points — there are more than 1,000 traditional acupuncture points — is related to different organs and regions of the body and is believed to affect their functioning. According to traditional Chinese medicine, each meridian has a starting acupuncture point and a terminal acupuncture point, which is connected to the starting acupuncture point of another meridian. Thus all the meridians of the body are interconnected, creating an endless cycle of "free-flowing energy."[9] Treating a starting point will affect the entire length of the meridian; that is, the direction of the flow of energy along a meridian remains constant after flowing through the point of entry.[10]

Acupuncture, itself not fully explained as yet, is believed to work at least partly by diverting or blocking the electrical signals which inform the brain that something in the body is hurting. The pain signals just don't make it through the system to the brain where the pain is perceived. The addition of magnets to acupuncture needles may improve their efficacy by increasing the amount of current they generate. It is a reasonable leap of faith, therefore, to suggest that the magnetic field itself generates tiny electric currents as parts of the body move through it — again, the Faraday effect at work. Even the blood flowing through the magnetic field may be enough to induce low levels of electric currents between or within blood cells. If any such currents are generated, they may well have the same effect as acupuncture does, namely blocking or diverting the pain-signaling electric impulses.

At the same time, of course, there are many other forces that may be at work in producing acupuncture's undoubted efficacy in preventing and reducing pain. Some of these may also help to explain the efficacy of magnet therapy. It is believed that acupuncture decreases pain by encouraging the release of endogenous opioid peptides (see chapter 6 for a further explanation of these), since pain relief achieved by acupuncture can be reversed with naloxone, an opioid antagonist.

Still, the similarities between magnet therapy and acupuncture are distant. They depend on the assumption that part of the mechanism whereby magnets reduce pain is that they activate electric currents, and thus replicate to an extent the current created by acupuncture. While the theory is certainly plausible, it remains somewhat tenuous. The reason for some doubt is that acupuncture works because, over centuries of trial and error, its practitioners have learned where many of the electricity-conducting passages are to be found; however, the application of magnetism — even where fixed magnets are attached to certain body parts — is far more generalized. In other words, the analogy between magnetism and acupuncture may provide a clue as to how magnetism works, but not much more than that.

However, there may yet be another explanation as to why acupuncture and, by analogy, magnetism work. By connecting the blood supplies of two rabbits in a cross-circulation pathway, one researcher showed that acupuncture stimulation of one rabbit inhibited the pain-related behavior in the other. This suggests that a blood-borne substance might be involved in the effects of acupuncture,[11] which could be activated by both acupuncture and magnetism.

MAYBE IT STIMULATES THE BRAIN DIRECTLY

Another way magnets may work is to stimulate the nerves of the brain directly. This effect can be observed easily enough when large doses of *electromagnetic* stimulation are applied. For example, an article by Drs. Mark Hallett and Leonardo G. Cohen in the *Journal of the American Medical Association* refers to a substantial body of work indicating that, in many cases, magnetic stimulation can replace the far more invasive and painful use of electricity to stimulate nerves. The authors point out that "the results of magnetic stimulation of the brain are similar to those of electric stimulation." Thus it can be used in many cases where the more traditional method has been electric current: for example, with Bell's palsy, a facial nerve disorder that causes twitches and disfigurements.[12]

The uncontested fact that electromagnetic stimulation of the brain can affect the nerve-carried electrical impulses in very much the same way as directly applied electricity does not necessarily mean that permanent magnets can achieve the same result. Nevertheless, it seems reasonable to assume that, at least up to a point, this is exactly what they do.

Indeed, the work done by Dr. M. J. McLean and his colleagues, first in 1991 and then (in more sophisticated form) in 1995, has largely verified this theory. Using a strong magnetic field (much stronger than the field emitted by therapeutic permanent magnets currently on the market), the researchers studied mouse neurons in a cell culture. Although this type of research is subject to the criticism that it is purely theoretical and hardly applicable in practice, the findings are instructive because they suggest that exposure to a permanent magnetic field causes the sensory neurons to change their electric behavior. They do so in a way that indicates that if the same effect could be induced in a living creature, a reduction in pain would be a likely outcome.[13]

Unfortunately, this particular theory of how permanent magnets work is inconclusive. So far, we know only that permanent magnetic force does *something*. That means that, proven or not, it is entirely likely that what it does could have a significantly salutary effect on many of the types of headaches, such as migraines, that are known to be correlated with a perturbation of the brain's electrical currents. We know that the effect of electromagnetism on migraines is often very dramatic. Thus the expectation that a substantial benefit can also be obtained from permanent magnets, and that the mechanism by which the magnetism works is similar in both cases, is not unreasonable.

OR MAYBE IT AFFECTS THE PINEAL GLAND

Yet another possible theory, and one we feel has at least as solid a basis as either of the electrical-stimulation theories, is that a magnetic field can work on the pineal gland and so induce a cascade of effects on all sorts of biological outputs, including the production of melatonin, serotonin, and various enzymes. Such changes could, of course, have a major impact on our ability to sense pain.

The fact that the pineal gland is strongly affected by *electromagnetism* has been very clearly established. Few researchers would doubt that today. Nor would most researchers doubt that the pineal gland affects many pain conditions, including, for example, migraines. Supporting his conclusion with 20 closely reasoned, research-backed arguments, Dr. Reuven Sandyk proves beyond reasonable question in his 1992 article in the *International Journal of Neuroscience* that "collectively, the data indicate an association between migraine headache and alterations in pineal melatonin functions."[14] This is a classic scientific understatement. In fact, the data *prove* his point.

What Sandyk does not prove, however, is just how this impact on the pineal is achieved. At least one research team, led by Dr.

A. Lerchl of the University of Texas, feels that the impact of electromagnetism on the pineal is not direct, but rather derives from "induced eddy currents resulting from the rapid on/off transients of the artificially applied magnetic field." It is those eddy currents, not the electromagnetism itself, that Lerchl believes reduce the production of melatonin and increase serotonin.[15]

Even though the effect of an electromagnetic field on the pineal gland seems unarguable, the theory that a similar effect may occur with permanent magnetism is still in the speculative stage. One adequately conducted study on rats showed no change in the pineal gland or in the rats' body chemistry when weak permanent magnets (810 gauss) were placed in their cages. As the investigators pointed out, however, "Studies such as ours result in permanent magnetic fields that are nonhomogeneous and difficult to measure as the animals move about."[16] Clearly, these results are not conclusive, especially since the Weinberger study on synovitis in rats cited in chapter 3 showed pretty definitively that the painful joint inflammation that characterizes that disease was greatly suppressed. Perhaps the difference between the two tests was merely that the synovitis one used a stronger magnetic field (3,800 gauss). More probably, the effect of increasing blood flow — which, as previously noted, is a major benefit of magnet therapy — may be more important to suppressing synovitis than changes in body chemistry are. In other words, as in so many instances in highly complicated modern medicine, the jury is still out.

THEN AGAIN, MAYBE IT'S BECAUSE . . .

Several other theories, interesting to speculate about, but with only limited experimental backing, are being discussed in the scientific community at present. It has been postulated that magnetic fields may partially realign certain molecules in the membranes of our cells, thereby distorting the conductivity (technically, the "ion-specific channels") enough to alter their behavior. Dr. Isadore Rosenfeld in his *Guide to Alternative Medicine* describes how Robert Holcomb, a professor at Vanderbilt University, used his electron microscope to show Rosenfeld that placing small magnets on selected parts of the body altered the orientation of the chromosomes within cells. Holcomb is convinced that this shift in position of the chromosomes leads to relief of acute and chronic pain. As a result of these observations, Rosenfeld, too, takes magnet therapy for pain very seriously.[17]

A more easily understood and, perhaps, more plausible explanation is that permanent magnetism inhibits the buildup (or reduces already existent) cholinesterase, an enzyme in nerve endings that tends to inactivate acetylcholine, a chemical that is essential to pain control. This theory was tested recently at the University of Tokyo. Using guinea pigs, the researchers compared the effect of permanent magnetism to the pained muscle, and needling to the acupuncture point. Since the animals could not describe their pain levels, the investigators did it for them by measuring what is called their "twitch response." The results showed that all the techniques, to varying degrees, reduced pain (or at least the pain as indicated by "twitch height"). The researchers then went on to try to determine why this happened. In reviewing the effect of magnetism, they injected the animals with a chemical that inhibits cholinesterase, and found that the result was exactly the same as from the magnets.[18]

Of course, that doesn't prove the magnets work in the same way; the similarity in results could be a mere coincidence. It is,

however, an interesting hint, and, incidentally, yet another indication that permanent magnetism works to reduce pain, even if we are
not quite sure how.

Finally, there is yet another reason why permanent magnetism may work. In a sense, this phenomenon, while not fully
explaining why magnetic fields affect pain, is most persuasive in explaining why they do *something*.

As most schoolchildren who have studied chemistry or even
earth science know, magnets *ionize* dissolved salts such as sodium
chloride, or common table salt. That is to say, they separate the positive ions of sodium from the negative ions of chlorine. Now, if you
can demonstrate this simple physical phenomenon in the lab easily
enough, it seems reasonable to suppose that a similar ionization
process could take place in the body, which contains quite a number
of dissolved salts. Of course, the degree of ionization would be very
limited, both because the magnetic force is minor and because only
one pole is in contact with the body at one time. But some sem-
blance of such a phenomenon could well be occurring, and it could
have an effect on how we feel pain.

Lonny J. Brown, PhD, reminds us that according to a principle of physics called the Hall effect, which has been around for a
hundred years, the positively and negatively charged ions in the
bloodstream become active when passing through a magnetic field,
and produce heat. The effect is to dilate the surrounding capillaries
and promote an increased supply of blood, which delivers nutrients
and oxygen and removes waste products and toxins more efficiently.
He also recognizes that other biologic elements, including elec-
trolytes, iron, the pH balance, hormone production, and enzyme
activity, may also play a role in our overall healthful response to
magnetism.

The fact is that while each of these theories may have some validity, none is wholly conclusive. Of course, it is possible that none of the currently existing theories on *how* magnets work is correct. A completely different explanation may emerge before long.

"Why does it matter?" you may well ask. Are we simply trying vainly to count the proverbial angels dancing on the head of a pin?

If we knew exactly the mechanism by which permanent magnetism worked, we believe we would be able to improve and refine our application of it. As it is, our knowledge is empirical. We can show that permanent magnetism works, but not yet exactly how. In time, and probably not too far in the future, more will be known about the subject — and we will be all the more effective at maximizing the efficacy of permanent magnets. (As new information comes to light, it will be made available on Brenda Adderly's website at www.BrendaAdderly.com.)

Chapter Six

MEDICATIONS:
PAIN RELIEF AT A PRICE

It's an ache; no, it's a throbbing; no, it's a burning sensation; it's always there; no, it comes and goes like a pulsing. Who can say which description of pain is accurate? As we were preparing to write this chapter, a woman said to us, "I don't envy you. I know where and when I experience my pain, but I have difficulty describing it, let alone writing about it." That is likely true for most of us.

Pain. How do you define it? We suggest that although it is a universal experience, a reliable description nevertheless remains elusive.

The word *pain* derives from the Latin *poena* and the Greek *poinē,* which mean "penalty" or "punishment"; the most ancient understanding of pain was as punishment for offending the gods.[1] Indeed, many modern people with poor self-esteem sometimes feel that their pain is no more than they deserve. For some persons, especially those who have experienced an injury, pain can involve a complex constellation of feelings of guilt, loss, and punishment.

The International Association for the Study of Pain has made an attempt to define pain, describing it as "an unpleasant sensory and emotional experience associated with actual or potential tissue damage."[2] Doesn't help much when you're in pain, does it?

There are probably as many other definitions of pain as there are authors who write about it. Like the preceding one, most of them are inadequate or irrelevant for the person experiencing pain, for if pain is anything, it is definitely a subjective experience, difficult to express and difficult to quantify.

Its intensity and the way we respond to it are not just dependent on actual physical damage, but are often related to our perception of, and emotional response to, pain. For instance, we can frequently change the intensity of our pain just by deliberately focusing our attention on it, and often can reduce its intensity when we are concentrating on something else. Persons who "catastrophize" (make every situation a major disastrous and negative one, no matter how insignificant) cope less well with pain.[3]

Our experience of pain also depends on our emotional state, how energized or depressed we feel, and even the influence of past training. Perhaps your mother told you as a child, "Don't complain about every little pain." And you still don't today, giving your pains scant attention or gritting your teeth and struggling through even when, perhaps, you should attend more to certain pains.

A NOTE ON PAIN THRESHOLD

Your tolerance for pain — your recognition of the first barely perceptible pain — will definitely affect the way you respond to pain. In the laboratory, pain threshold is measured as the lowest intensity that will cause pain.

Pain-threshold studies use mechanical methods of producing pain — pressing on certain particularly sensitive areas, applying pressure with some sort of gauge, inflating a sphygmomanometer cuff (blood pressure cuff) to the point of pain, applying heat or cold — to determine the factors that influence our perception of pain. Largely an experimental concept, it *has* helped shaped our understanding of clinical pain.

Laboratory studies have found 27 different factors other than analgesics that produce variation in the pain threshold, but different studies often arrive at conflicting results. Still, some generalities do exist. For instance, pain perception and attitudes about pain and pain relief apparently differ according to culture. Women appear to have a lower pain threshold than men, although studies here are not consistent. One British study found that back pain was substantially more common in women over age 55 than in men of the same age.[4] A review of pain studies found that while women reported more severe levels of pain, more frequent pain, and pain of longer duration than men did, women also are much more proactive than men in finding solutions.[5]

Pain threshold tends to rise with age. Mental fatigue, fear of pain, and anxiety can all lower the pain threshold for some people. Distraction raises the pain threshold, as does a placebo when the recipient expects relief. The side effects of some drugs (nausea, peripheral vasoconstriction, respiratory depression) alter pain threshold. Pain perception can vary between the dominant and nondominant sides of the body. Increased experience of pain in childhood likely results in greater sensitivity to pain as an adult.[6]

False information can also affect a person's report of pain. Two studies performed to assess the relationship between estimates of subjective pain and the actual pain stimulus were conducted at the University of Texas. For the 20 subjects, subjective estimates of pain with no feedback rose with the increasing pressure of a blood pressure cuff. In another session, numbers ostensibly reflecting cuff pressure were shown on a slide. Even though the numbers did not always reflect the pressure accurately (some were higher, some lower), pain ratings were higher during high-feedback conditions and lower during low-feedback conditions.[7]

HEADACHES: THE MOST COMMON PAIN

Headaches are the most common recurrent medical complaint in the United States. They account for 1.7 percent of all primary care office visits; more than 40 million Americans have headaches severe enough to require medical attention. Between 65 and 80 percent of people suffer at least one significant headache annually, and half of those will have one or more severe headaches a month.[8] Sometimes our prescription medications — especially appetite suppressants, oral contraceptives, estrogens, and blood-pressure medications — cause our headaches.[9] For others, daily headaches may result from caffeine or medication *overuse.*

In a relatively new category of headache, the chronic daily headache, analgesic abuse is a common problem. When 220 patients attending a headache clinic in Thailand were examined, 60 (27.3 percent) were diagnosed as suffering from chronic daily headache. More than half of that group consumed analgesics on a daily basis.[10] Reviews of headache patients throughout the world indicate the incidence of analgesic-induced headaches ranges from a low of 2.3 percent of all headaches to a high of 60 percent. About 1 percent of the German population takes up to 10 pain tablets daily. It has also been calculated that the adults living in the urban areas of Modena, Italy, take an average of 15 mixed barbiturate-analgesic tablets, or 18 packages of mild analgesics, per year.[11]

Although headache specialists have known about it for a long time, the "rebound" headache is just now appearing in the literature. Persons who take medications too frequently or in excessive amounts often experience a decrease in therapeutic efficacy. A cycle of increased consumption secondary to increased pain develops, whereupon the analgesics not only do not cure headaches, but actually intensify them. This paradoxical effect is called an analgesic-induced headache, or a rebound headache.[12] We know of at least one popular acetaminophen product — and we are sure there are others — that is renowned for causing rebound headaches. The more you take the product for headaches, the more headaches you continue to have. Talk about a built-in market . . .

On the other hand, patients consuming analgesics daily for diseases other than headache seem to develop daily headaches only at a rate ranging from 2 percent to 5 percent.[13]

Rebound headaches also occur when patients who have habitually overmedicated themselves on aspirin, acetaminophen, and other analgesics abruptly discontinue them. The situation makes it difficult for the physician to prescribe other analgesics or condone the use of over-the-counter drugs for relief of the headache,[14] and often adjunctive methods have to be taught for pain control (see chapter 8). The doctor in the know, however, might simply "prescribe" magnets, or the patient might enlighten his doctor about them.

Lest you think headache and other pains are largely diseases of the aging or those who overuse medication, you may be surprised to learn that the highest prevalence of headache, backache, muscle pain, and stomach pain is found in the 18-to-24 age group.[15]

Pain will always be with us. It is one of the universal conditions all persons experience at some time in their lives and, often, one of the hardest to describe and to understand. Aristotle described pain as one of the "passions of the soul." It has likely been "a major clinical problem since the beginning of medicine,"[16] and pain control remains "one of the great problem areas of contemporary medicine in spite of many years of intensive research."[17]

DOESN'T EVERYONE FEEL THE SAME WAY?

Although pain frequently signals an abnormality or a specific danger to our well-being, individuals' attitudes toward pain are not uniform. Often they are shaped by religious faith, our particular society's attitude toward suffering, or by other influential aspects of our upbringing. For instance, a prominent television commercial by a well-known pharmaceutical company suggests that the modern-day hero is one who has "challenged" his pain and won by taking its brand of pain pill.

Two studies carried out at Duke University Medical Center indicated that undergraduates who had a strong family history of pain problems reported a greater number of pain sites and higher levels of pain-related interference with activities.[18] A study carried out in Sweden with 148 men between the ages of 45 and 55 showed that an individual's perception of the strenuousness of a physical workload, as well as beliefs that his task was too difficult or presented too great a responsibility, were more prevalent in men with intermittent or chronic low back pain.[19] A Swiss study revealed a statistical trend for low job autonomy, high job demands, and low job satisfaction to be related to back pain for men. Among women participating in the study, dissatisfaction with salary was the only work-related factor associated with back pain.[20]

While your own pain and how you control it may seem intensely personal, in the larger and more worldwide sense pain and pain relief are intimately intertwined not only with our individual personalities and personal belief systems, but also with morality (shape up or we'll hurt you or let you continue to hurt) and ethics (one kind of pain will be allowed and relieved, another kind will not). Nurses may bring preconceived ideas and expectations about the kind and amount of pain associated with various diagnoses to their treatment of patients, and may have problems dealing with patients who don't conform to those expectations.[21]

The influence of medical, social (family estrangement/divorce), and economic (loss of a job due to pain, the cost of pain management) values of the world's societies affect attitudes toward pain as well. Many elderly people accept pain as a part of the aging process, failing to come forward for medical help, while for others complaining about pain is seen as a very effective form of communication with their family or caregivers.[22] Studies have documented the statistical association between childhood psychological traumas and the development of chronic pain disorders in adulthood.[23]

One expert has called pain a "learned experience." By this he means that our reactions — what we think the sensations mean, what we consider appropriate behavior when the pain has been identified, and what response we can expect from ourselves and other people — have all been learned from our life experiences and training.[24]

In 1969 a British doctor coined the term "illness behavior" to refer to those actions a person shows to the world in response to a medical situation.[25] When the illness behavior is proportionate to the level of disease present (as determined by a doctor, of course), the behavior is considered "normal." When patient complaints or symptoms go beyond what can usually be expected from a specific disease process (also determined by a doctor), the behavior is commonly considered to be "illness-affirming," whether it is engaged in consciously (as in malingering) or unconsciously (as in pain where psychological factors are presumed to play a central role).[26]

ACUTE VS. CHRONIC PAIN

Pain specialists divide pain into two categories: *acute* and *chronic*. The therapeutic management of them is quite different, although one of the traps for patients with chronic pain, and sometimes their doctors, is in using an acute-pain model rather than a chronic one.[27] It has been estimated that in the industrialized countries, 15 to 20 percent of the population have acute pain and between 25 and 30 percent suffer from chronic pain.[28]

Statistics from the National Health Interview Survey of 1995 show that 13.7 percent of the U.S. population were limited in activity in some manner due to chronic pain conditions, and approximately 9.3 percent of the population experienced limitation in major activities. By the end of the century, it is likely that 18.2 percent of the population of the United States (37.9 million people) will go to their doctors with arthritic complaints.[29]

Think of it. During their lifetime, one in three U.S. citizens experience some form of chronic pain that requires medical attention.[30] Chronic pain is often so subtle a condition that diagnosis is difficult, and treatment may emphasize the patient–physician relationship.[31]

Acute pain has a recent onset, usually within the last seven days, and usually results from a specific event or accident, although its origin can be unknown. Acute pain typically starts near an area of the body that has been damaged, and the pain serves the biological function of warning that something is wrong that needs to be taken care of. It is less likely than chronic pain to have psychological components, although it is possible. Some believe that acute pain is related more to anxiety and chronic pain to depression.[32]

Historically, narcotic analgesics have been the mainstay of treatment for acute pain, especially for acute postoperative pain.

When our bodies receive relief from acute pain, they usually get busy with healing, and the use of pain medication is relatively brief, although extensive tissue damage can extend the duration of time that someone requires pain medication.

Pain that last more than six months, sometimes with an unknown origin, constitutes *chronic pain.* One doctor goes so far as to describe chronic pain as a "malefic force" that can impose severe emotional, physical, economic, and social stress on everyone involved: the person in pain, his or her family, and even society.[33]

According to one primary care physician, chronic pain most often comes in the form of headache, low back pain, nerve injury, myofascial syndrome (pain that originates in one muscle or its fascia, but is felt in another location), and facial and oral cavity pain.[34] Others believe that chronic pain often has lost its function as a symptom of an underlying medical condition and that *the pain itself has become the "disease."*[35]

Although narcotics are often effective for acute pain, they are usually contraindicated for chronic benign pain because of the risk of addiction. One pain management specialist believes that the use of narcotics interferes with pain management and rehabilitation of the typical chronic pain patient — one study showed that more than 50 percent of patients abused prescription analgesic medications — but that if they *are* going to be used, there needs to be a well-defined structural lesion, psychological and social factors need to be minimal, and there should be no history of previous alcoholism or addictive disease.[36]

While the etiology of acute pain is almost always known or can be readily discovered, chronic pain is frequently believed to be based on a complex interaction of physical and psychological factors, and the debate rages as to what these are and how important they are. The old division of pain into organic and psychogenic (no physical cause) has been replaced. Most doctors no longer tell patients that because they can't find something structurally wrong, their pain is all in their head. Still, certain psychological factors can be involved in any kind of pain, but especially chronic pain.

A profile of the chronic pain patient who is least likely to benefit from opioids is someone who has poorly defined specific pain, has no identifiable structural problem, and is frequently unemployed. He or she has often seen multiple physicians and is likely to be receiving workers' compensation or other forms of disability payments. This kind of patient has a "pain-centered lifestyle."[37] Some would disagree with this description. An evaluation of the psychological state of more than 4,000 patients who suffered low back pain and sciatica found that only 5 percent had psychopathy. However, in a comparative group of more than 2,000 chronic pain patients, most of whom suffered low back pain, 75 percent had personality dysfunction and antecedent psychiatric disease. While displaying less physical impairment than the larger group, they nevertheless suffered more disabling symptoms.[38]

Patients who experienced noncardiac chest pain during exercise but who lacked cardiac ischemia (localized tissue anemia due to obstruction of the inflow of arterial blood), as determined by nuclear scanning, were compared to patients who had both ischemia and chest pain and patients having neither. The family histories and psychosocial problems of the three groups differed considerably. The noncardiac-chest-pain patients had the highest levels of parental divorce, personal psychiatric treatment, current depression, somatic awareness, anger control, and negative attitudes toward the health care system.[39]

Doctors may need to consider a person's attitude toward

pain and suffering before chronic pain can be resolved. Habits a person has developed to cope with his or her continuing pain may actually aggravate it, and relief may depend on the person's developing more effective coping procedures, such as learning to breathe differently, taking relaxation and/or visualization breaks, and, of course, using magnets.

The outcome of the attempts to manage chronic pain can be affected considerably by the expectations of both the doctor and the patient. The Australian psychologist Rosemary McIndoe says that chronic pain patients, and sometimes their doctors, carry "chronic pain myths," which may have to be dispelled for effective treatment. Some of those include "hurt means harm to the body," "real pain is organic," "search long enough and you will find the cause and the cure," and "you have to learn to live with it."[40]

Before you get the idea that all chronic pain patients have deep-seated psychological problems that influence their progress, we want to assert that there is a group of chronic pain patients who have mild to moderate pain, do appear to have a structural disease, have minimal disability, and no psychological problems. They do well with low doses of narcotics, which allow them eventually to return to work. A third group also has the preceding characteristics but their pain does not seem to be amenable to therapy. They, too, do well on larger doses of opioid analgesics,[41] and might do even better using magnets. In fact, magnets might relieve their pain sufficiently to let them reduce their analgesics or get off them completely.

HOW THE BODY NATURALLY
ATTEMPTS TO SUPPRESS PAIN

In the last two decades, clinical research has contributed a great deal of information about pain through experimentally creating acute pain and its relief. Although pain may begin at a particular location, it has to travel through the nerve fibers of the spinal column to the brain for us to "feel" it.

If we were to slice the spinal column across horizontally, we would observe that the center part is roughly in the shape of a butterfly. We call the back part of the butterfly's wing the posterior horn, and many types of nerve fibers that transmit pain to the brain are in that horn. The brain, however, can also send its own signals to the horn that encourage it to fight pain.

One of the more accepted theories of how this works is called the *gate control theory*. Its publication in 1965 kindled a new interest in pain treatment and research; the researchers who worked on it won a Nobel Prize.[42] The gate theory suggested for the first time that pain control might be achieved by enhancing normal physiological activities, as opposed to the previously popular idea of surgically cutting so-called pain pathways in the spinal cord.

Put most simply, gate theory is based on the concept that transmission of nerve impulses from peripheral areas of the body to the spinal cord can be blocked by a gatelike mechanism in the dorsal horn of the spinal cord. The theory proposes that the cells in the posterior dorsal horn, or cells in the nucleus of cranial nerve V, act like a gate to increase or decrease the flow of nerve impulses from peripheral fibers to the brain. Ronald Melzack and Patrick Wall, the originators of the theory, proposed that the dorsal horn has two kinds of fibers that conduct pain: thick or large fibers (inhibitors) and small or thin ones (facilitators). Thick fibers conduct stronger impulses, and conduct them faster, so when pain signals from the fibers meet, the stronger signal suppresses the weaker. Thick-fiber inputs tend to close the gate, whereas thin-fiber inputs generally open it and cause pain.

While the gate control theory has generated considerable research, controversy, conflicting evidence, and revision, in many circumstances it remains a popular way of understanding how pain messages get to the brain.[43] As a result of the gate theory, researchers found that selective activation of large fibers by direct or transcutaneous (meaning "through the skin") electrical nerve stimulation (TENS) to the skin produced relief from a variety of pain states, including low back pain and myofascial pain. The actual TENS procedure involves placing two electrodes (that are attached to a power source) on the skin over the area of pain. While the exact mechanism of how this type of electrical pulse therapy works is still not known, it seems to be most effective for those localized musculoskeletal pains that are unrelieved by NSAIDs (nonsteroidal anti-inflammatory drugs) or mild analgesics. The amount of time necessary to teach successful TENS utilization often results in its being more frequently used to treat chronic rather than acute pain.[44] Therefore, with acute pain, you may be able to achieve similar results using your magnets.

A second wonderful discovery that altered the way the medical world viewed pain treatment was the 1973 discovery, by Dr. Candace Pert and her colleagues, of specific binding sites in the brain for opioids, and discoveries in subsequent years that the body produces chemicals or peptides (endogenous opioids) that activate those opioid receptors. Now lumped into the general category of endorphins, the first of the endogenous opioids, the enkephalins, was announced in 1974 and the detection of beta endorphin followed the next year.[45] Later studies revealed that each opioid receptor arises from its own gene and their primary effect is to reduce neurotransmission.[46] Dynorphin, the most recently discovered endorphin, is thought to be 10 times more potent a painkiller than morphine.

The endorphins are another of the body's natural ways to block or kill pain, and they do this by attaching themselves to the opioid receptors of a cell. Two researchers have suggested that the presence of opioid receptors in our bodies may be related to an "endogenous pain-allaying mechanism" that permits injured prey to escape from a predator.[47]

Several researchers have reported that baseline endorphin levels are lower than normal in chronic pain patients, and that electrical stimulation at acupuncture points increases their levels.[48] One of the problems with the long-term use of narcotics is they have a tendency to reduce our body's natural production of endorphins. The more narcotic painkillers you use, the less ability you have to produce endorphins. Therefore, some physicians think that TENS is ineffective for patients who are simultaneously taking narcotics, while the use of drugs that activate the action of endogenous pain-suppressing transmitters may improve the effectiveness of TENS.[49]

PAIN BEHAVIOR: OUR RESPONSE TO PAIN

Many pain therapists refer to the differences in people's perception of pain and the way they respond to it as "pain behavior." This is not to say that you don't have "real" pain, but that, as we said earlier, how you experience pain — its intensity or regularity, for instance — may be influenced by social and psychological factors.

Although clinical evidence is inconclusive as to the relationship between personality traits and pain behavior, one British researcher found that, in Britain at least, while introverts appear to be more sensitive to painful stimuli, they express their pain less freely than extroverts.[50] The more introverted you are, the lower your pain tolerance is.[51] Mothers in labor who were classified as introverts felt pain sooner and more intensely than extroverts, complained less, but tended to remember the pain more vividly afterward.[52]

Two studies of undergraduate students conducted at Duke University Medical Center found that the number of reported pain sites was significantly higher for women than men, and that women were more likely than men to report that pain interfered with their activities.[53] However, it's never quite clear in gender studies whether the difference between men and women is that women actually experience more pain or that men are less likely to admit they have a pain problem.

The hazards of trying to reduce pain relief to a purely physiological problem and leave it, often unsuccessfully, at that have led many pain management programs to adopt a holistic approach to pain relief, wherein more factors than just the simple fact of pain, and its relief by analgesics, are considered.

F. M. Alexander, the Australian actor who developed the Alexander technique of movement, also coined the term *end-gaining,* which refers to the desire to go after a goal without paying attention to how it is reached, without being engaged in the process. End-gaining does not permit us "to be open and flexible to possibilities, to be inclined to see what unfolds."[54] It's easy, using magnets, to ignore information about the "emotional process" that may be occurring along with the pain. So don't forget, while you're using your magnets for pain relief, to be open to the possibilities of the emotional factors or attitudes your pain may be expressing. You will have to attend to them for ultimate pain relief.

ANALGESICS

Medications or drugs that control pain without a loss of consciousness are called *analgesics*. They can be further divided into *narcotic* and *nonnarcotic* pain relievers.

Among the nonnarcotic analgesics we can include the nonsteroidal anti-inflammatory drugs, or NSAIDs, and stimulation-induced analgesia (SIA), produced by acupuncture and certain devices like TENS units that electrically stimulate various parts of the nervous system or brain. British humor suggests that NSAID really stands for "nearly [the] same [as] aspirin in disguise,"[55] but it isn't so.

The trick in pain relief is to find the right medication or procedure for the individual, while doing as little damage to the body as possible and encouraging the cooperation of the person as much as possible. You'll see that becomes almost a magic trick, or perhaps an illusion, as we delve into the side effects of analgesics. To further complicate the issue, one doctor advises that when maladaptive behavior coexists with chronic pain, nonnarcotic analgesics, NSAIDs, and tricyclic antidepressants are seldom effective *by themselves* in resolving the pain.[56] We have to add more medication, with more possible side effects. Time to head for the magnets.

NONNARCOTIC ANALGESICS: NSAIDs

Nonnarcotic analgesics are the most frequently purchased over-the-counter medications. They are the object of an annual outlay of millions of dollars by the American public. It's astonishing to consider the extent of their use. Various reports estimate that between 13 million and 17 million patients in the United States take NSAIDs, and these drugs have become the mainstay in the first-line medical treatment of osteoarthritis, rheumatoid arthritis, and other rheumatologic disorders.[57] A number of NSAIDs are administered by prescription only — more than 90 million prescriptions for NSAIDs are filled annually in the United States,[58] but we will limit our discussion to the more common kinds of NSAIDs — ones you have likely purchased over the counter in the past, or may even have in your medicine cabinet now.

NSAIDs are big business. Unfortunately, that business comes with its own built-in set of problems for users. A large portion of the people who purchase these pills don't realize that they have potential toxic effects.

NSAID therapy is associated with upper gastrointestinal symptoms in 25 percent of patients and causes ulcers or erosions in 40 percent of patients with long-term use, and lower gastrointestinal complications in 10 to 15 percent of users. If we take the top estimate of NSAID users, 17 million, this translates to 100,000 to 200,000 ulcer complications. One doctor estimates that side effects from NSAID use results in 10,000 to 20,000 deaths each year.[59]

The Reuters news service reports that according to the Arthritis, Rheumatism, and Aging Medical Information System, approximately 76,000 people are hospitalized each year for gastrointestinal complications caused by chronic NSAID use. The estimated annual cost for treating these patients is around $760 million.

Given all this trouble, what is it that NSAIDs do that makes them so popular and useful? Put most simply, pain from tissue injury occurs both as a direct result of injury to nerve endings and by inflammation secondary to the release of chemicals from the nerves and damaged tissue. More specifically, with the onset of almost all forms of tissue damage, the body releases certain prostaglandins (fatty acids that produce hormonelike actions) at the site of the damage. They sensitize the body's pain receptors, called nociceptors, which exist throughout the body in skin, viscera, blood vessels, muscle, and fascia (connective tissue). Their sensitization by the prostaglandins increases the pain response to chemical mediators such as histamine and bradykinin that are also released when a cell is damaged by trauma. The release of all these proinflammatory agents also sensitizes adjacent nociceptors, resulting in an increase in the spontaneous activity of some nociceptors and alerting the body to potentially damaging stimuli.[60]

By using NSAIDs to inhibit or block the synthesis of prostaglandins, activation or stimulation of the pain receptors is reduced and pain perception is decreased. As you've learned, NSAIDs predominantly do their job at the site of an injury to inhibit the initiation of pain impulses, rather than in the central nervous system, where opioid or narcotic drugs principally act.

This makes NSAIDs especially helpful in controlling minor or moderate pain, such as that experienced with headache, toothache, and low back pain. As their name implies, they are most effective in providing relief for pain associated with inflammatory conditions, which usually occurs where the prostaglandins, particularly prostaglandin E2 and prostacyclin, have done their work. Although NSAIDs reduce the swelling of inflammation, their effects may not be seen for several days in severe cases.[61]

Generally all NSAIDs have analgesic effects, but they may vary considerably in their anti-inflammatory activity and many contain other ingredients such as antacids or caffeine. You've probably used such combinations. They include Alka Seltzer, Anacin, Comtrex, Coricidin, Dristan, Excedrin, Midol, Sinarest, Sinutab, Vanquish, and many other over-the-counter products.

NSAIDs Plus Antidepressants

When used as analgesics, the NSAIDs have a ceiling; that is, a dose beyond which further improvements in pain reduction will not occur.[62] Their overall analgesic effect often can be enhanced by using them in conjunction with other medications, such as opioid analgesics or tricyclic antidepressants, the latter being helpful for persons in whom depression is an important component of their response to pain, or whose depression is giving rise to pain. A historical review of the literature indicates, however, that patients with low back pain, fibrositis (a rheumatic disorder of fibrous tissue), and fibromyalgia (a chronic musculoskeletal condition characterized by diffuse musculoskeletal pain, aching, poor sleep, and fatigue) do not show significant improvement when antidepressant drugs are added.[63] They do improve with magnets.

Further, tricyclic antidepressants are not without their own set of problems, especially for elderly patients with cardiovascular disease who may experience such adverse effects as arrhythmia (irregular heartbeat), congestive heart failure, and urinary retention. When taken by the elderly, confusion states may also develop. Common side effects of antidepressants include dry mouth, blurred vision, constipation, sedation, appetite stimulation/weight gain, impotence, excessive drowsiness, and precipitation of glaucoma.[64] All cyclic antidepressants can lower seizure threshold and need to be avoided by those with a history of seizures.[65]

It's not clear why the antidepressants work in pain relief. Their effectiveness may be related to the fact that their psychotropic activity alleviates accompanying anxiety and depression, or to an ability to exert a direct analgesic action, or to the potentiation of the analgesic activity of other drugs.[66] Pain patients who benefit from antidepressants often report pain relief before feeling any uplift in mood, leading to the speculation that the antidepressant works by increasing the supply of the neurotransmitter serotonin.

When used as part of a combination drug regime, lower doses of all the medications can often be used, reducing potential side effects, but not necessarily the time it takes to achieve pain relief. One doctor estimates that 80 percent of all prescription analgesics sold or promoted in the United States are a combination of analgesic drugs, with aspirin being the single most common denominator.[67]

Aspirin

Salicylates (aspirins such as Bayer, Empirin, Norwich) are among the most commonly used NSAIDs. In an article commemorating the centennial of the synthesis of a shelf-stable form of acetylsalicylic acid by Felix Hoffmann of the Bayer Chemical Works in Elberfield, Germany, on August 10, 1997, *Newsweek* reported that some 50 billion doses of aspirin are consumed annually worldwide.[68]

The effectiveness of salicylates was known more than 2,000 years ago, when Hippocrates used the bark of the willow tree (genus *Salix*) for relief of pain and fever.[69] At the time of Hoffmann's discovery, Bayer, basking in the sales of its newest product, heroin, didn't get around to marketing aspirin for another two years.[70]

Because of its effectiveness and relatively low cost (when compared to prescription NSAIDs), aspirin is often used as a first line of defense in inflammatory conditions.

After ingestion, the salicylates are absorbed by the stomach and the upper parts of the small intestine. It is not unusual, then, that common side effects of the salicylates include stomach upset and gastrointestinal bleeding. For some, aspirin use causes ringing in the ears, loss of hearing, and various allergic reactions (rashes, itching).

Overdose can lead to severe diarrhea, fast breathing, drowsiness, and convulsions. Prolonged or excessive use of aspirin forces the kidneys to excrete more vitamin C and potassium, causing a depletion of these nutrients.[71] Prescription aspirin combinations that contain narcotic drugs certainly have the potential to create narcotic dependence when taken on a continuing or long-term basis. Low-dose aspirin, however, is clinically proven to reduce the risk of heart attack.

Adults who are at risk for adverse reactions to aspirin include those with allergies, ulcers, anemia, bleeding disorders, asthma, high blood pressure, and kidney or liver disease. Because it can promote excessive bleeding, aspirin should not be used in the days before or after surgery, including tooth extraction.[72]

A number of NSAIDs have become available since the discovery of salicylates, but many of them are no more effective than aspirin and considerably more expensive. Their use should be, but is not necessarily, confined to patients unable to take aspirin due to gastrointestinal side effects or to individual hypersensitivity.

Ibuprofen and Naproxen

Ibuprofen (Advil, Motrin, Nuprin), a derivative of propionic acid, is another popularly used NSAID, especially for mild musculoskeletal pain. Although ibuprofen has a lower incidence of side effects when compared with other NSAIDs, it also has only weak anti-inflammatory action.

Common side effects that accompany the use of ibuprofen include stomach upset, gastrointestinal bleeding, heartburn, dizziness, and drowsiness. Less common side effects that have occurred are intestinal gas, constipation, and loss of appetite. Overdose signs include lethargy, low blood pressure, difficulty breathing, and irregular heartbeat. People with diabetes, asthma, kidney or liver disease, colitis, ulcers, congestive heart failure, and high blood pressure are at high risk for adverse side effects when they use ibuprofen.

Another propionic acid derivative is naproxen (Aleve, Naprosyn, Anaprox), frequently used for osteoarthritis, rheumatoid arthritis, bursitis, and gout. Its side effects and high-risk groups are generally the same as ibuprofen's. In addition, for some people its use may result in photosensitivity, the development of skin rashes or painful irritation when exposed to sunlight.

The gastrointestinal side effects of NSAIDs — which may occur because they interfere with prostaglandin formation necessary for stomach mucosal maintenance — cannot be ignored. One doctor estimates that in Canada, more than 2 percent of patients followed for five years were at risk of developing peptic ulceration from the continued use of NSAIDs.[73]

When 174 patients with chronic low back pain were divided into three groups, one of which received NSAID therapy in combination with spinal manipulative therapy and supervised trunk exercises, the NSAID group did no better after five and eleven weeks than the other two groups, which received combinations of spinal manipulative therapy combined with trunk-strengthening exercises or the exercises alone. All three groups improved, and it was the continuance of exercise during the follow-up year, regardless of type of therapy, that resulted in a better outcome for pain reduction.[74]

Acetaminophen

Acetaminophen (Actamin, Tylenol, Valadol) technically is not an NSAID, but is often discussed or included with them. Although uses for acetaminophen have been known since 1893, it did not come into widespread use until the mid-1940s.

Acetaminophen is useful for persons who cannot tolerate aspirin and can be found under more than 150 different labels and as an active ingredient in more than 200 proprietary drug combinations.[75] It is also useful for treating mild pain, and is a widely used adjuvant to opiates for severe pain.

A major advantage of acetaminophen products is that they do not cause gastric irritation and have a minor effect on blood coagulation. This makes acetaminophen useful for those who have bleeding disorders or are taking oral anticoagulants. Because acetaminophen causes only minimal inhibition of peripheral prostaglandin synthesis, it is considered a weak anti-inflammatory agent and not as effective in treating inflammatory conditions such as rheumatoid arthritis.[76] The toxic dose of acetaminophen is lower than for aspirin, so overdose is more dangerous; acute overdose or even chronic use can cause severe and sometimes fatal liver damage.[77]

Other Drawbacks of Using NSAIDs as Painkillers

All analgesics have the potential to cause changes in the body beyond the reduction of pain. Some analgesics will result in heightened sensitivity to the drug with prolonged use, eventually requiring less medication or a change in medication. As a person ages, his or her sensitivity to analgesics can increase. In general, older persons become more sensitive to, and suffer from, the side effects of NSAIDs more frequently than younger adults.[78] If the person continues to imbibe "standard" doses, or takes them on a time schedule derived from the use of the drug on younger persons, the likelihood of adverse reactions increases. NSAIDs have been cited as provoking approximately 20 percent of all the adverse drug reports filed with the Food and Drug Administration.

Long-term use of some analgesics can effect changes in liver and kidney functioning. Although acetaminophen and aspirin can alleviate postoperative pain, they also suppress fever, which may mask an infection. High dosages or long-term use of acetaminophen can result in liver toxicity, while continued use of NSAIDs can result in platelet dysfunction.[79] NSAIDs also cause asthma attacks in about one-fifth of all asthmatics.[80]

One study showed the incidence of gastric ulcer in patients receiving aspirin to be 18 percent, while the duodenal ulcer rate was 4.6 percent.[81] Females, elderly persons, and patients with previous ulcer disease who take pharmacologic doses of steroids, or have concurrent debilitating disease, or who use alcohol or tobacco are most susceptible to NSAID-induced gastric complications.[82]

When autopsies were conducted on the bodies of 713 patients, 249 of whom had had some form of NSAID prescribed during the six months before death, significantly more (21.7 percent) ulcers of the stomach or duodenum were found in those who had used NSAIDs than in those who had not. Further, more NSAID users than controls (N = 464) had two or more ulcers (controls were persons for whom NSAIDs had not been prescribed during the six months before their deaths). Three patients (4.1 percent) out of the group who were defined as long-term users (N = 74) of NSAIDs (NSAIDs other than aspirin prescribed daily for six months preceding death) had died from peritonitis resulting from perforated non-specific small intestinal ulcers. Long-term users had more ulceration and perforation of the small intestine, while the short-term NSAID group (NSAIDs prescribed daily for less than six months or discontinuous courses of NSAIDs prescribed for six months or more) had more gastric ulcers.[83]

While the gastrointestinal and renal side effects of NSAIDs are well known, less recognized is the potential for cardiovascular toxicity, including exacerbation of hypertension and congestive heart failure, especially in the elderly.[84]

In summary, some of the many adverse effects associated with NSAIDs include:

1. gastric irritation, dyspepsia, even ulceration leading to hemorrhage (specific gastric irritation can often be controlled with the addition of another medication)

2. diarrhea or constipation; nausea and vomiting

3. sodium and water retention, which may precipitate cardiac failure in persons with heart disease

4. reduction in renal blood flow, which may lead to a reduction in urine production; kidney failure in persons at high risk of renal damage

5. acute bronchospasm, urticaria (a skin allergy), and edema, particularly in some persons with chronic obstructed airways disease, a history of asthma, and nasal polyps; they may also be at increased risk from the respiratory-depressing effects of NSAID and opioid drugs

6. reduction of platelet aggregation and prothrombin, which is what makes low doses of aspirin useful in preventing strokes and heart attacks

7. tinnitus (ringing in the ears), diminished hearing, vertigo (dizziness), hyperventilation; in extreme cases of overdose,

mental confusion, seizures, hallucinations, and even coma, primarily from high levels of aspirin taken over time

8. liver dysfunction, in rare instances; it is usually reversed when the medication is discontinued

9. reduction of iron in the blood

10. bleeding (when taken along with oral anticoagulants), low blood pressure (with diuretics), loss of antihypertensive effect (with various blood pressure drugs), toxicity and bone marrow damage (with methotrexate), inability to control voluntary movements and other features of central nervous system toxicity (with lithium).[85]

Because of the many possible side effects of NSAIDs, and their continued popularity, nondrug techniques, such as weight reduction and strengthening of supporting muscles for musculoskeletal pain, should accompany, and help minimize, their use.[86]

NARCOTIC ANALGESICS: OPIATE/OPIOID DRUGS

Some of the most common narcotic analgesics are those classified as opiate/opioid. As soon as they were discovered, narcotic analgesics became one of the medical profession's greatest assets. Their effectiveness is as undisputed as the problems and adverse effects they cause. For instance, while most effective in producing pain relief after surgery, many of them also produce respiratory depression (slowed-down breathing), nausea, vomiting, constipation, dizziness, and sometimes an addictive euphoria. All the opioids act directly on the central nervous system. Continued use over time may result in dependence or addiction to the drug, as well as a decrease in a person's natural defenses against pain and stress.[87]

Originally *opiate* was the term applied to drugs such as

morphine and codeine that were obtained from the opium compound. In its natural state, opium is derived from the dried juice of the unripe heads of the poppy *Papaver somniferum,* commonly called the "opium poppy." When pharmaceutical companies developed the ability to synthesize drugs with morphinelike action, such as methadone, meperidine (Demerol), and propoxyphene (Darvon), the term *opioid* was developed, and now is frequently used as a generic term for any natural or synthetic substance that binds to opioid receptors and reduces pain.[88]

In its various forms, opium is the most widely used narcotic analgesic. Common opium derivatives include morphine, codeine (methylmorphine), methadone (Physeptone, Amidone), and a number of other drugs used before, during, or after surgery, such as papaveretum (often used before surgery) and phenoperidine (frequently used as an adjunct to anesthesia).

The most common side effect of, and fear about, long-term use of opioids for pain relief is the development of dependence or addiction. Therefore, many pain management texts advise against using them for low back pain, in spite of the fact that a review of more than 60 articles in the medical literature revealed no controlled studies that indicate chronic opioid analgesic therapy (COAT) is inappropriate for persons with chronic low back pain. In fact, case reports on a total of 566 patients suggested that COAT was safe and effective for many patients with recalcitrant chronic low back pain. Nevertheless, the review authors suggest that preexisting substance abuse, certain personality disorders, certain medical conditions, and certain occupational factors are contraindications for employing COAT. They also suggest that along with the administration of COAT, treatment should include contracts, family interviews, and continued monitoring for drug problems until the time when patients achieve some relief. Then an exercise regimen should be initiated.[89] In other words, there's no free ride; no long-term use is appropriate.

Increasing tolerance (shorter periods of relief requiring more frequent use) results in a need to use more and stronger doses and may result in dependence or addiction. The degree of physical dependence and the time required to develop it vary greatly with individual agents.

While dependence is not likely to develop during the short-term use of narcotics for acute or postoperative pain, it frequently develops in the majority of patients who need to take regular opioids for longer than three to four weeks. When the narcotic is no longer needed, in order to reduce withdrawal symptoms its discontinuance may require slow detoxification by progressively decreasing doses, or the introduction of another narcotic such as methadone or clonidine, rather than abrupt cessation.

Drowsiness is a common feature of opioid use, although occasionally some opioids have mood-elevating or euphoric effects. They also suppress the cough centers in the brain, resulting in less coughing (remember codeine cough syrup?), which can be helpful for critically ill patients who require tracheal intubation (a tube in the throat) for help in breathing.

Opioids slow down emptying of the intestines and can lead to spasms of the anal sphincter, resulting in constipation, or contraction of muscles in the bladder and urinary sphincter, causing difficulty in urinating. Large doses can release histamines, resulting in itching and urticaria.

The most significant undesirable effect of opioids, especially for cardiac patients, is respiratory depression. Morphine may also produce nausea and vomiting, although chronic use may suppress the vomiting center. Chronic morphine use also decreases the functioning of the adrenal cortex, and inhibits the secretion of the thyroid-stimulating hormone and the pituitary growth hormone.[90]

Barbiturates, nonbarbiturate sedatives, and tranquilizers are other commonly prescribed drugs, although as the addictive quality of barbiturates has become widely known, physician prescriptions for them have gradually been declining. Barbiturates cannot relieve pain without impairing consciousness when used alone for pain. Elderly persons are particularly vulnerable to sedatives and narcotics. With advancing age, their ability to absorb the drugs is affected in a variety of ways, depending on the drug used.

Morphine given intravenously to the elderly in the usual adult dosage has been known to cause symptoms of severe toxicity. Some think this may be due to older patients' decreased liver and kidney functions; others suspect the elderly may have fewer opioid receptors. Either way, this means that even a small amount of a narcotic drug is likely to have a more pronounced effect.[91]

USING PAINKILLERS RESPONSIBLY

Not only budget-wise but health-wise, it pays to be careful about the painkillers you use and to know their specific side effects. If you can't understand the printed descriptions of a drug that many pharmacists provide with your pain-relief prescription, ask your pharmacist for the specific side effects. Combining the use of narcotics with alcohol, skeletal muscle relaxants, or mood-altering drugs (tranquilizers, tricyclic antidepressants, MAO inhibitors) can result in a number of untoward reactions, most notably intensifying the narcotic's depressant effect, possibly with fatal results.

If you use adjunct therapies such as biofeedback or relaxation techniques in your pain management program, as you learn to relax more quickly and deeply you may require a lower dose of your pain medication and run the risk of overdose if you aren't knowledgeable and vigilant. The same is true for magnets. If your use of aspirin, for example, has become automatic (you *know* you need to take two aspirins every four hours because you've done it for months, even years), you certainly may be overdosing if the use of adjunctive techniques, including magnets, reduces your pain. We know that for some people, magnets seem to work right away, and they don't need to take their nonprescription drug habitually. For other people, magnets attain effectiveness more slowly. During this time you may wish to gradually reduce your regular pain medication to allow the magnets to achieve maximum pain relief and to enhance your awareness of your body's reactions. Certainly if you are on a prescribed pain medication, ask your doctor or pharmacist about reducing its use gradually and whether there are any side effects to that process.

Pain relief from using either NSAIDs for prolonged periods or magnets may allow persons to increase their activity. We know this is exactly what you want, and that you believe it is desirable at all times, but in some instances increased activity can cause you to overuse an already stressed joint with implications for damage or more pain in the future. So while you may be able to move without pain once you have strapped on, or otherwise affixed, a magnet to your pain site, don't immediately jump up and engage in such vigorous activity that you impose stress on a damaged or inflamed joint.

We hope this chapter has aptly demonstrated why magnets may be a preferred choice over common pain medications in some instances. The next chapter will provide some helpful hints on their use.

Chapter Seven

HOW TO USE MAGNETS TO TREAT YOUR SPECIFIC PAIN

Currently most experts agree that the way to use magnets is quite simply to put them over the sites that are causing pain. What makes the difference is the strength of the magnet.

Most of those little kitchen magnets you have on your refrigerator won't work; they aren't strong enough. The permanent magnets used in treating pain vary in strength from about 300 gauss (for magnets in some shoe insoles) to 3,950 gauss (for many common types of pain, including low back pain), to even more. Some are disc-shaped, some are rectangular. They are usually held in place by adhesive tape, state-of-the-art support braces, or Velcro wrappings. The magnets themselves usually weigh less than two ounces. Thus, while worn, they are hardly noticeable. The fact that so many Senior PGA golfers wear them while they compete attests to their unobtrusiveness. In terms of how long the magnets should be worn, there is no definitive guideline, although several hours tends to be the norm, regardless of the type of pain. Many people choose to wear them longer, and some only when engaged in a strenuous activity.

Dr. Whitaker learned firsthand about the therapeutic use of magnets from one of his patients, Jackie I. Jackie lives in Alabama but has been coming to the Whitaker Wellness Institute in Newport Beach, California, twice a year since the mid-1980s. At the time of her first visit, her blood pressure was out of control, and she had constant lower back pain. Diet changes, a regular exercise program, and a comprehensive nutritional supplement program enabled Jackie to get off blood pressure medications and live more or less pain-free for the next ten years, with only occasional flare-ups in her back.

However, about a year ago, Jackie's back pain returned with a vengeance. She was unable to walk, and the lack of exercise was driving her blood pressure up. A friend brought over a thin, pliant magnet about the size of a videocassette and showed her how to place it over her lower back. By the next day she noted pain relief, and within a week she was able to resume her 45-minutes-a-day walks. She felt so much better with this magnet that in addition to wearing it on her back every day, she also began wearing magnetic insoles in her shoes and sleeping on a magnetic mattress and pillow. She claims to sleep better, wakes up completely rested, and has more energy than she has had in years. Her blood pressure is back to normal, without medications.

Other doctors attest to similar results. Dr. Charles W. Kennedy, Jr., head of Orthopedic Associates of Corpus Christi, the largest orthopedic group in South Texas, became interested in magnets after his wife developed tennis elbow in her right (dominant) arm. It did not respond to a combination of physical therapy, exercise, cortisone injections, and NSAIDs. She was scheduled for surgery, but after considering the length of the scar and the unpredictability of success, Mrs. Kennedy resigned herself to future discomfort — until someone told her about magnets.

Mrs. Kennedy wrapped a band of magnets around her forearm just below the elbow. Two and a half weeks later, she was without pain, and the Kennedys became converts, so much so that Dr. Kennedy has now become the president of MAGNAflex Inc., a company developed to assist manufacturers and distributors in North America in taking services, equipment, and technological developments in health care into Mexico. The company's second intent is to "take biomagnetic therapy through the FDA" via scientific studies. It has already arranged for the first Institutional Review Board double-blind study of magnet therapy, which has been completed by Baylor Medical School in Houston and has been accepted for publication by *Archives of Physical Medicine and Rehabilitation,* a nationally recognized, peer-reviewed journal. (At the time of the writing of this book, the study had not yet been released.)[1]

Like Dr. Whitaker, Dr. Kennedy is not only an advocate for magnet therapy, but a user as well. For occasional low back pain resulting from a degenerative disc, he often wears a 4-by-6-inch magnetic pad against his lower back and experiences an almost immediate decrease in pain. He states he has effectively used magnets with his patients for various conditions, including tendinitis, carpal tunnel syndrome, low back pain, anterior knee pain, and more. According to Kennedy, the advantages of magnet therapy are that it is extremely cost effective, noninvasive, and in those cases that are successful, there is an almost immediate decrease in the amount of discomfort.

SAFETY PRECAUTIONS

Although many agree that, unlike drugs, magnets have no side effects, there are some safety precautions we recommend.

First, persons with pacemakers and insulin pumps should not use them, because of the possibility that magnets might interfere with the magnetically controlled features of these devices.

Second, since the effect of magnetism, if any, on fetuses is unknown, women who are pregnant should not use them.

Third, because of the belief (still unproven) shared by many that magnets work by dilating the blood vessels, and thus get more blood flowing into the area that's in pain, until further studies are conducted we advise against using magnets immediately after a sprain. Theoretically, doing so might increase the amount of hemorrhage into the area. However, an interesting case study presented on the use of permanent magnets to speed up postoperative healing showed much promise, as the magnets used in that study were reported to have markedly reduced postoperative bruising.[2]

Until more studies are conducted and reported, ice down such injuries to reduce swelling and inflammation, and immobilize the area for a day or two before applying magnets. Also, since you wouldn't want to increase the blood flow of a fresh wound, until more studies are conducted magnets should not be applied immediately to such injuries either.

Finally, people undergoing treatment by transdermal drug delivery systems (patches) should not wear magnets close to the patches. If the theory that a magnet increases blood flow is correct, then conceivably the magnet might also cause more of the drug to enter the bloodstream within a shorter period of time than intended. It's unlikely that a magnet placed on the lower back would interfere with a patch worn on the chest, for example, but err on the safe side and do not place a magnet over or within the same anatomical area as a patch.

COMBINING MAGNETS WITH ACUPUNCTURE POINTS

Scientists are becoming aware that the cell membrane is more than a protective shield studded with receptor sites. They are beginning to understand that it is a powerful signal amplifier or interactive window through which the cell can sense and respond to its minuscule environment. It allows some substances to pass freely back and forth and acts as an impenetrable barrier to protect the cell from intrusion by other substances.

When designated molecules flow into special receptor sites, a subtle signal produces a sudden change in electrical tension between the exterior and interior of the cell, and for a few thousandths of a second the barrier opens, producing an atomic- or molecule-size channel or passageway.

We suggested in chapter 5 that one possible explanation for the effectiveness of acupuncture is that the needle inserted in the skin generates a small electrical current, that twirling the needle may cause the current to pulse, and warming it may slightly increase the strength of the current.

Many believe that in addition to the receptor sites for chemical stimuli that cell membranes have, they also have similar sites for subtle energy signals. Or perhaps not so subtle. In spite of the prevailing Western view at the time that if acupuncture worked at all, it worked through the placebo effect, Dr. Robert O. Becker and Maria Reichmanis, a biophysicist, showed that most acupuncture points possess greater electrical conductivity than other points in the body, and, further, that the meridians were conducting current.[3]

Electrical stimulation of highly specific areas in the pain pathway produces relief just as effectively as microinjections of morphine, and the effects of acupressure anesthesia can be reversed by the use of antimorphine drugs. If we *combine* amounts of morphine or electrical stimulation that alone are too weak to reduce pain, we still produce relief. This suggests that weak electrical stimulation relieves pain by acting at specific receptor sites in a manner identical to that of morphine. (Morphine binds to the opioid receptors mu, delta, and kappa in the brain.) Furthermore, the specific locations that permit molecular or electrical signals to relieve pain are precisely the sites of action of the endorphins. In other words, acupuncture releases endorphins, or naturally occurring morphines, into the nervous system. With this discovery, the status of acupuncture changed from a "quack" procedure to one more readily accepted by Western medicine.

Similarly, it seems likely that static magnetism can work effectively on acupuncture points. We therefore recommend the following procedure: First try placing the magnets directly on the sites causing pain. If that relieves the pain, keep using them in that way. If not, try adding them to the acupuncture points as discussed below. (Remember also to keep in mind the importance of stress management, proper diet and exercise, and following any traditional treatments prescribed by your doctor.)

The first step in combining magnets with acupuncture (and acupressure) concepts is, of course, to determine the places on your body where you experience pain. Then, in addition to putting the magnets over the areas causing pain, also place them over the nearest acupuncture point above and below the area of pain. Dr. Kennedy believes that the combination of placing magnets over the site of pain and over acupuncture points results in a "logarithmic increase in effect." Use figures E–J to determine where those acupuncture points are.

REFERRED PAIN

Dr. Ronald Melzack and his colleagues have spent a great deal of time investigating the effects of acupressure. An interesting bit of Melzack's work involves myofascial pain or referred pain, which is pain that originates in one skeletal muscle or its fascia (connective tissue), but is felt in another location. Its originating site can be

COMMON ACUPUNCTURE POINTS

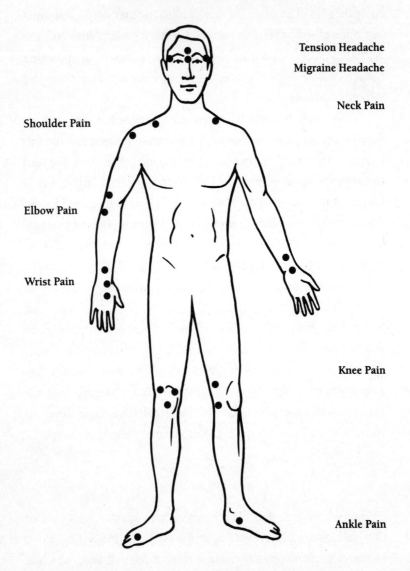

Figure E. Acupuncture point references courtesy of Vicki Weissler, OMD, L.A.c.

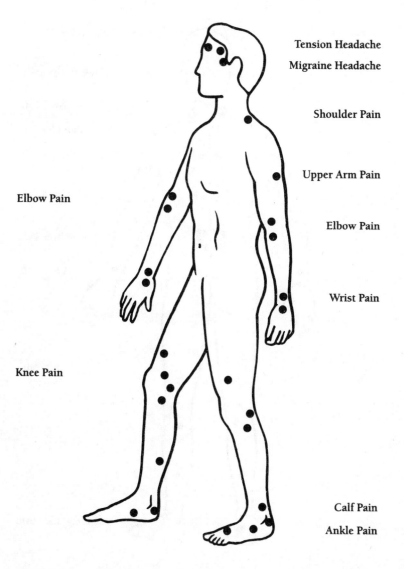

Figure F.

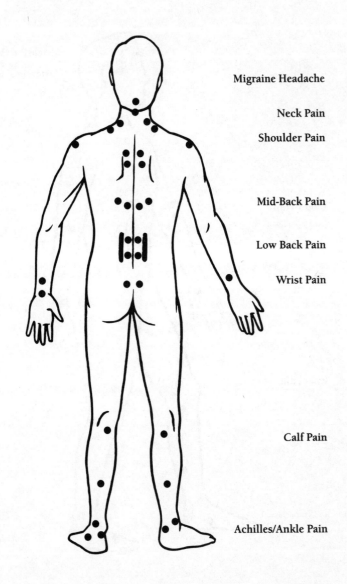

Migraine Headache

Neck Pain

Shoulder Pain

Mid-Back Pain

Low Back Pain

Wrist Pain

Calf Pain

Achilles/Ankle Pain

Figure G.

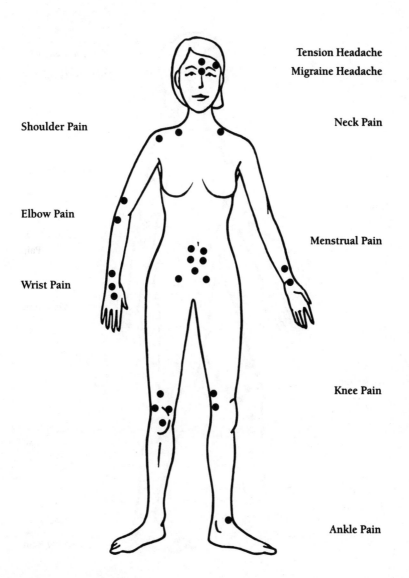

Figure H.

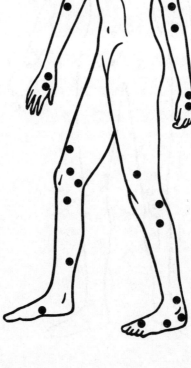

Tension Headache

Migraine Headache

Shoulder Pain

Upper Arm Pain

Elbow Pain

Elbow Pain

Wrist Pain

Knee Pain

Calf Pain

Ankle Pain

Figure I.

HOW TO USE MAGNETS TO TREAT YOUR SPECIFIC PAIN

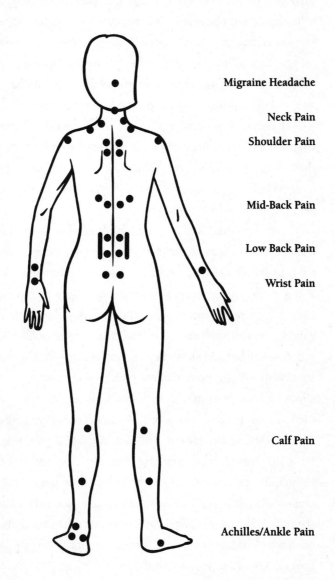

Migraine Headache

Neck Pain

Shoulder Pain

Mid-Back Pain

Low Back Pain

Wrist Pain

Calf Pain

Achilles/Ankle Pain

Figure J.

identified by pressure on tender trigger points, which elicits a pattern of pain felt elsewhere and specific to particular trigger points. Myofascial trigger points, especially those in the neck (sternocleidomastoid), head (temporalis), and upper back (trapezius) can be significant contributors to the etiology of chronic tension headaches.[4]

Referred pain follows specific patterns based on the 32 original segments, or dermatomes, of our embryonic development. One trigger point in the neck can send pain into your hand because the dermatome at that location includes not only the neck but also the lower portion of the forearm, half the palm, and the three outer fingers.[5] Who would have thought it?

It is believed that an initiating stimulus — such as soft-tissue trauma, blows, sprains, fatigue, stress, poor posture, overuse patterns in sports and occupations — causes a physiological response that generates a "hyperirritable locus," or trigger point. Once sensitized, trigger points can cause such muscle maladies as stiffness, fatigability, weakness, and restricted range of motion. The painful muscles may become shortened and cause pain when stretched. Persons with trigger points often protect their painful muscles by adopting poor posture with sustained muscle contraction, which in turn may cause the development of additional trigger points.[6]

Some of the earliest work on myofascial pain was done by Dr. Janet Travell, who, working from her own review of Chinese techniques of acupressure, identified trigger points to treat the chronically ailing back of President John F. Kennedy. At that time, she treated the trigger points with passive stretches and injections of anesthetic. Today myofascial therapists apply pressure with their fingers, knuckles, elbows, and specially shaped bars or wooden shafts, called bolos, to break up the spasm at the trigger point before using gentle stretches and movements to help reeducate the muscle to stay relaxed. Without the stretches, it's likely that stress will activate the trigger points again.

Dr. Melzack found that every trigger point reported in the Western medical literature has a corresponding acupuncture point,[7] which means that sometimes you may want to try putting your magnets over the trigger point in order to relieve a pain that you actually experience elsewhere. If magnets alone do not resolve the pain, you may also want to try the combination of acupressure (pressure on the acupuncture point) and magnets, both on the trigger point and on the acupuncture point nearest the pain. Figures K–P show prominent trigger points that may cause pain in the referenced areas.

COMMON TRIGGER POINTS

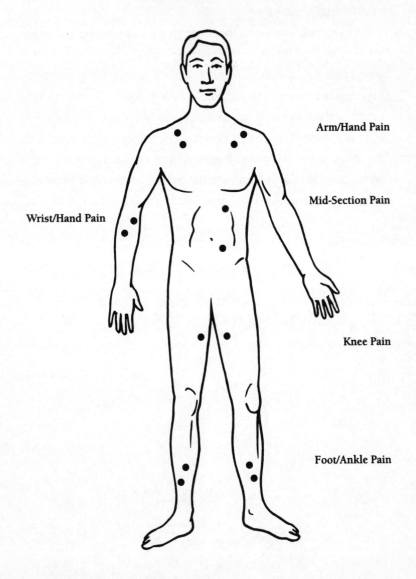

Arm/Hand Pain

Mid-Section Pain

Wrist/Hand Pain

Knee Pain

Foot/Ankle Pain

Figure K. Trigger point references courtesy of Robert Mueller, Ph.D., Ms.T.

HOW TO USE MAGNETS TO TREAT YOUR SPECIFIC PAIN

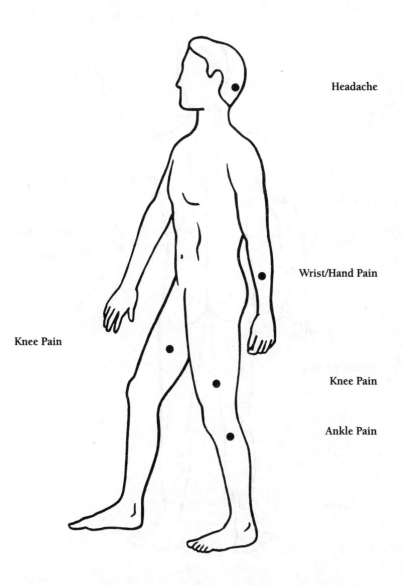

Headache

Wrist/Hand Pain

Knee Pain

Knee Pain

Ankle Pain

Figure L.

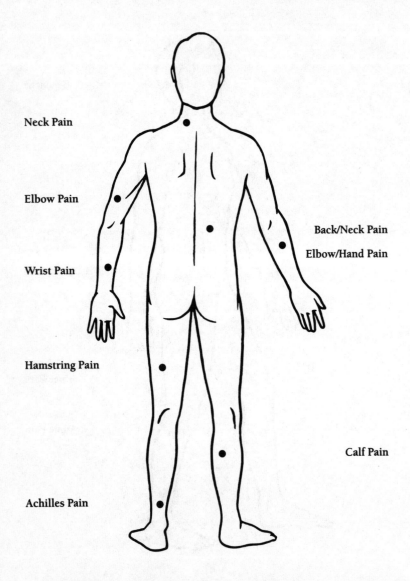

Neck Pain

Elbow Pain

Back/Neck Pain

Elbow/Hand Pain

Wrist Pain

Hamstring Pain

Calf Pain

Achilles Pain

Figure M.

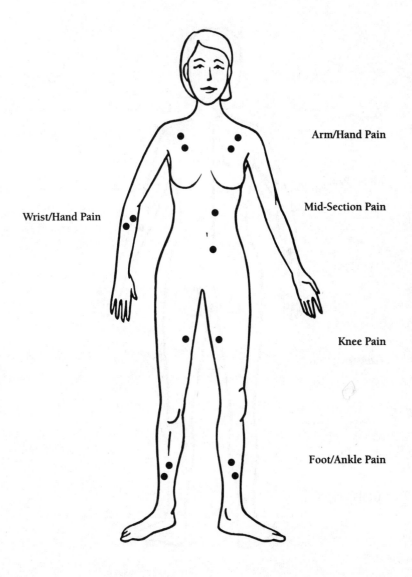

Arm/Hand Pain

Mid-Section Pain

Wrist/Hand Pain

Knee Pain

Foot/Ankle Pain

Figure N.

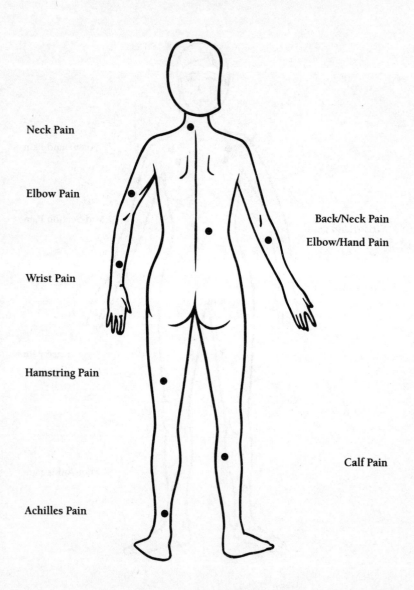

Neck Pain

Elbow Pain

Wrist Pain

Hamstring Pain

Achilles Pain

Back/Neck Pain

Elbow/Hand Pain

Calf Pain

Figure O.

HOW TO USE MAGNETS TO TREAT YOUR SPECIFIC PAIN

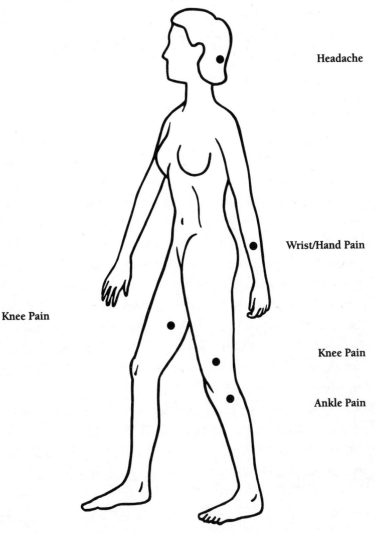

Headache

Wrist/Hand Pain

Knee Pain

Knee Pain

Ankle Pain

Figure P.

Chapter Eight

EXERCISE THAT HELPS, NOT HURTS

"I don't want to move when it hurts," you say. And we understand; sometimes we feel the same way. But common sense, the experience of many people who don't move when it hurts, and the literature on exercise programs clearly show that it is *not* moving that gives you stiff muscles, muscles that will also hurt the next time you try to move them.[1] Too often people don't exercise because they erroneously believe that exercise will automatically aggravate a painful condition and that rest cures chronic pain.[2] The opposite is true, however. It is motion that promotes healing in the musculoskeletal system. Lack of motion leads to stiffness, cartilage degeneration, and muscle atrophy.[3] Magnets can get you back into the swing of things by relieving pain so you'll feel like exercising.

Not only does inactivity cause you to hurt more and feel worse, it runs counter to what the psychiatrist Adele Pace says is our "innate appetite for physical activity." Exercise triggers the production of dopamine and other pleasure-giving neurotransmitters. When we work out regularly, the brain comes to crave this rewarding bath of messenger chemicals.[4] Exercise also helps the body burn off undesirable levels of catecholamines, the breakdown products of adrenaline, which are released by the body during stress reactions.

"I'm too tired to move" is another excuse we frequently hear for not exercising. The fact is, however, that in many instances exercise can give you the energy boost you're looking for. Fatigue may actually be caused in part by a lack of exercise. Experts call this "sedentary inertia," or sometimes "energy deficiency." Antidote? Movement, which the Australian psychologist Rosemary McIndoe suggests might be a better word, since the word *exercise* seems to frighten some people in pain.[5] Research is also beginning to accumulate that shows that seniors with sleep complaints rate their sleep quality as improved after initiating a regular exercise program of moderate intensity.[6]

The Surgeon General's 1996 Report on Physical Activity and Health found that 60 percent of all American adults don't get the recommended amount of exercise and 25 percent aren't active at all, which may be, in part, why magnets are more appealing than a long-term approach. People with arthritis and other rheumatoid conditions are even less active, and this may have disastrous consequences for them. A four-year study of musculoskeletal impairment in a group of otherwise healthy adults (373 men and 259 women, average age 42 years) showed a general trend toward acceleration of musculoskeletal impairment of about 10 percent a year. Women showed greater increases in pain or discomfort. For both sexes, the most vulnerable anatomical locations were lower back, neck, and knees.[7]

On the plus side, some researchers have observed that participants in an exercise program who are in the poorest physical and/or psychological condition often show the greatest improvement not only physically but also psychologically.[8] So there's hope for even the most inactive among us.

The key lies in your attitude, in finding ways to enjoy your workouts, and in giving up the old idea that exercise is painful or boring, or that you're too old or too out of shape to exercise.

Change those messages to ones that help you anticipate exercise with pleasure. After all, Senior Olympian Edith Mendyka ran 100 meters in under 20 seconds when she was 70 years old, and swimmer John Fleck set a record for the seniors' 100-meter freestyle at the ripe young age of 99. What if they had said, "I'm too tired," or "I'm too old"?

A substantial part of what we think of as age-related decline in physical capabilities is actually due not so much to aging as to decreased and insufficient physical activity.[9] Doctors at the Veterans Administration's Geriatric Research, Education, and Clinical Center in Gainesville, Florida, emphatically state that many of the diseases associated with age, and possibly aging itself, can be either treated or alleviated by an active lifestyle. Cardiac, pulmonary, musculoskeletal, and metabolic–endocrine declines associated with age and/or disease often show a change in progression as a result of increased physical activity.[10]

The research is clear. A huge body of scientific evidence illustrates that exercise is an important adjunct in the treatment of osteoporosis, heart disease, depression, osteoarthritis, rheumatoid arthritis, and fibromyalgia, to name just a few conditions. Exercise is especially useful in relieving pain. Let's look at the effects of exercise on perhaps the most common site of pain, the lower back.

EXERCISE AND LOW BACK PAIN

For acute low back pain, it may be appropriate at the onset of pain to use your magnets in order to maintain your ordinary activities rather than take to your bed. When city employees in Helsinki, Finland, with acute low back pain were assigned either bed rest for two days (67 patients) or back-mobilizing exercises (52 patients) and compared with a control group advised to continue ordinary activities "as tolerated" (67 patients), the control group had better recovery after 3 and 12 weeks than the other two groups. Moreover, the bed-rest group experienced greater duration of pain, pain intensity, and lumbar flexion, and had more days absent from work. As in many other studies, recovery was slowest among the patients assigned to bed rest.[11]

Most doctors and pain clinics agree that around 90 percent of patients with acute low back pain recover within a two-month period, irrespective of the type of treatment, and that while exercise probably does little to facilitate recovery from an acute episode, it is equally likely that it is an integral factor in preventing recurrent injury.[12] It pays to strengthen back and abdominal muscles to prevent another episode, since the recurrence rate is 40 to 85 percent within a year after the first incident, and that recurrence is characterized by increased frequency, longer duration, and greater disability.[13]

Ninety Finnish subjects with chronic low back pain were divided into three groups to participate in a three-month program. One group received intensive strength training, a second participated in home exercise, and the third was a control group. At the end of the three months and at an evaluation nine months later, both exercise groups experienced reduced intensity of back pain and improved muscular performance compared to the controls.[14]

There is an apparent contradiction between the clinical success of the commonly prescribed treatment of exercise to relieve low back pain and the disappointing results reported in the scientific literature. Further, while low back pain has been associated with both physically stressful and sedentary occupations, the literature on pain and exercise shows no clear association between low back pain and physical activity,[15] even though clinical and practical experience tell a different story. After all, how often have we heard a patient tell his doctor, "I hurt my back playing golf."

Some research evidence suggests that exercise in general is beneficial for *nonspecific* low back pain, yet inadequate study designs often make conclusions difficult. Further, there is lack of information in the professional literature about the types, frequency, and duration of exercises that should be prescribed and at what stage they are most helpful.

THERE'S STILL TIME TO MAKE A DIFFERENCE

Evidence is beginning to accumulate showing that it's never too late to begin a physical fitness program, provided you begin with a graduated program and work upward, finding the balance of movements and rest that works for you. Physical activity benefits the musculoskeletal system of people of all ages, has the potential to postpone or prevent some musculoskeletal disorders, and has even been shown to reduce the frequency of tension headaches.

Twenty patients treated for pain in a physical therapy clinic once a week for six weeks received education for posture at home and the workplace, an isotonic home exercise program, massage, and stretching of the cervical spine muscles. Their frequency of headaches decreased significantly and remained so during a one-year follow-up.[16]

It's likely that you may be able to move more than you think you can, and that your attitude and/or other social factors impose more constraints than your actual pain experience. Some researchers found, for instance, that when chronic pain patients performed their prescribed exercises "to tolerance" (as much as they

could before pain, weakness, or fatigue caused them to want to stop)
with machines that were altered so participants had no feedback as to time or the exact amount of exercise completed, the
amount of exercise performed increased steadily. Further, pain
patients did almost the same amount of exercise work as a control group of healthy young adults who responded to an advertise-
ment for an exercise program. Both groups did more work than a
previous reference group exercising with feedback. The researchers
conclude that our tolerance for exercise is often shaped or influenced by factors such as environmental reinforcement that are unre-
lated to pain.[17]

When patients with low back pain were requested to perform four exercise repetitions (two with each leg), it became apparent that expectations of pain were associated with a fear response
and an urge to avoid the pain.[18] Maybe you can move more than you
think, especially with the use of magnets: Dr. K. Mashima and his
colleagues have discovered that the lumbosacral joint is the most reliable "magneto-sensitive" part of the body.[19]

Furthermore, several studies show that exercise promotes an
analgesic effect. When 17 males who exercised on a regular basis
participated in 20 minutes of self-selected exercise and then rested
for 20 minutes, their pain tolerance (when pain was induced with a
gross pressure device) increased significantly after the exercise when
compared to their experience prior to exercising. The researchers
used self-selected exercise rather than a specified kind of exercise in
a controlled laboratory setting in order to show that the analgesic effect of exercise is possible in naturally occurring situations.[20]

When laboratory pain was induced by applying 3,000 g
force to the middle digit of the right forefinger for two minutes

before and after five minutes of cycling, the pain threshold was significantly higher and the pain ratings were significantly lower five minutes after the exercise condition compared with a condition of quiet rest for the same persons. The changes in pain perception in the exercise condition were also accompanied by lower systolic blood pressure and higher heart rate.[21]

A similar study was conducted with 60 males who were randomly assigned to either an experimental group, which exercised for 12 minutes by climbing a double step to recorded musical cadences, or a control group (no exercise). Results showed that exercise was a significant predictor of increased pain tolerance, as measured by the amount of time, up to 10 minutes, that the men could endure a 2,300 g pressure to the index finger of their dominant hand.[22]

HOW CAN I GET MOVING?

Why people who have been shown that exercise will reduce their pain don't continue to exercise is a great mystery to health care professionals. One study showed that belief in the benefit of exercise increased adherence, but a conflicting study found that both individuals who continued to exercise and those who did not believed exercise was helpful. For 110 people with osteoarthritis, a specific recommendation tended to increase their adherence, while a recommendation and printed materials were even better. Best yet, recommendations, printed materials, and physician monitoring increased adherence to 78 percent.[23] Apparently many of us need someone to keep track of us and give us positive feedback.

Ask yourself, What activities are important to you? What are your movement goals? What will you accept as reasonable or meaningful outcomes for your efforts? Can you be flexible in your adherence to your exercise routine? For instance, arthritis often has a fluctuating and sometimes unpredictable course. Instead of rigidly sticking to an exercise program, persons with arthritis who have learned to respond to changes in their symptoms can rationally adjust their exercise regimens.[24] You, too, can respond to changing levels of pain and stiffness, sometimes exercising less and using magnets more, sometimes applying your magnets for pain relief before or after you exercise. Be flexible mentally, and it may well be that your body will become more flexible.

Most comprehensive exercise programs focus on three goals: improving the cardiovascular system (aerobic movements), improving body strength, and improving flexibility. For each of these, you increase your exercise as your fitness improves, proceeding carefully and at your own pace. "No pain, no gain" is a motto that has lost credence, in general, and certainly has no place in your life. In fact, exercise that causes pain, and exercising while you are experiencing pain, can lead to severe injuries.[25]

AEROBIC TRAINING

The purpose of aerobic or cardiovascular training is twofold. It serves to improve the efficiency of your body in carrying oxygen from the air into the lungs and muscle fibers, and it improves the efficiency with which the muscles produce energy.

Cardiovascular training involves engaging in aerobic exercise with a goal of getting your heart rate into a "target zone" (50 to 85 percent of your maximum heart rate) and sustaining that rate for at least 20 minutes. The heart and circulatory system are best trained by continuous exercise that is slightly below your maximum capacity. By increasing the amount and the intensity of submaximal exercise, you increase your level of aerobic fitness.[26]

Common cardiovascular exercises include jogging, swimming,

bicycling, machine rowing, exercising on a treadmill, fast walking, in-line skating, and cross-country skiing. For many persons with chronic pain, especially arthritis, some of these activities may exacerbate symptoms, so choose your activity carefully. Swimming is the least likely to do so, and since it takes the weight off your lower back, it is a good exercise for people with low back pain.

Studies are beginning to accumulate that show the efficacy of aquatic exercise therapy in improving functional ability in a variety of disorders. Exercises and movement in a heated swimming pool where the gravity pull is reduced are becoming quite popular and effective for the relief of back, neck, and knee pain. Many YMCAs and YWCAs offer heated pools and some type of pool exercise program.

Where fear of falling limited the movement or exercise ability in elderly people, water exercises were found to increase their functional reach every week during a five-week "simple exercise" program. Land exercisers increased their functional reach only during the first week.[27]

When 13 subjects with rheumatic disease engaged in eight weeks of aquatic therapy, significant pre- and postexercise differences were found. The marked decrease in pain and in difficulty performing daily tasks contributed 94 percent to an overall increased functional status and active joint motion scores.[28]

Stair climbing appears to offer an advantage over treadmill walking for patients with claudication pain, which often accompanies certain arterial diseases. It is characterized by absence of pain or discomfort in a limb when at rest, but commencement of pain, tension, and weakness after walking is begun, progressing to the point where walking becomes impossible. Symptoms disappear after a period of rest.[29] Patients with peripheral arterial disease who are limited by claudication pain frequently have concomitant cardiovascular problems (hypertension, myocardial ischemia) during exercise. Although the times to onset and to maximal claudication pain as well as ankle systolic pressure did not differ between treadmill walking and stair climbing for 10 patients limited by claudication, their heart rate, systolic and diastolic pressure, and mean arterial pressure *were* lower during and following stair climbing. Stair climbing was well tolerated and safely performed by the patients and placed less demand on the cardiovascular system.[30]

Current recommendations for aerobic activity are for 20 to 30 minutes at least three days a week. You should aim to work at a level where you feel that your breathing is heavier but where you can still hold a conversation. If you're bored during aerobic activity, read, listen to an audio book, or listen to workout music.[31]

As with any exercise, warm up first for 5 to 10 minutes and cool down 5 to 10 minutes, in an activity at a lower intensity than the aerobic component — for example, take an easy walk or an easy bike ride.

To stave off boredom and maintain your interest as your conditioning improves, revise your goals upward. Cross-training, or changing to different kinds of exercise on various days, also helps keep interest high. Run on the treadmill or track on one day, swim laps the next, and use a regular or stationary bike on the third day.[32] While you're doing it, thank your stars you don't have to engage in the kinds of cross-training recommended by the third-century writer Philostratus for the early Greek athletes: endurance running, lifting weights, and wrestling with beasts, especially lions.[33] Still, that might serve to keep your interest high.

STRENGTH TRAINING

Evidence continues to mount that affirms the positive effects of strength training, or high-resistance exercise, for decreasing pain, for slowing the multiple losses of aging, and as an effective antidepressant. As you work with hand weights and/or weight machines, with gradual increases in the weights and the number of repetitions performed, you strengthen and firm your muscles (such as weak low back muscles), increase muscle mass, and increase endurance; that is, you build the capacity of the muscle to move for longer and longer periods of time — ultimately aiding your aerobic training. Strength training is also helpful when the cause of acute pain is trauma or tissue damage. It is generally accepted that an increase in venous return from the wounded area and an increase in blood supply to the area is therapeutic. Muscle activity facilitates both these actions.[34]

By reducing the changes in body composition that occur with aging — increased fat mass, decreased fat-free muscle, decreased total body water, and decreased bone density — strength training has been shown to raise the energy levels of elderly persons, and to increase their strength and functional capacity. These, in turn, reduce the risk for diseases such as non-insulin-dependent diabetes mellitus and osteoporosis.[35]

Strength training for the back and abdomen (when abdominal muscles are weak, the back is more susceptible to strain) helps reduce the incidence of low back pain. It also decreases the pain of osteoarthritis.

Ten people with osteoarthritis of the knee who participated in an eight-week program of muscle-strength training experienced a significant decrease in pain and stiffness, a significant increase in mobility, and a significant decline in arthritis activity compared to a control group. Three times a week the group completed six sets of five maximal contractions on a Cybex II dynamometer at 90 degrees per second.[36]

One doctor goes so far as to suggest that exercise and social support may be as effective as NSAIDs in reducing pain and improving mobility in persons with knee osteoarthritis and that treatment strategy should, therefore, change, using drugs only in an adjunctive role and only when exercise and social support prove ineffective.[37] A study conducted in Cape Town, South Africa, found that adding NSAIDs (either meclofenamate or dislofenac) to a standard physiotherapy treatment over a seven-day period did not improve the healing of acute hamstring muscle injuries. This was one time when the control group (physiotherapy but no medication) had a significantly lower level of reported pain at the end of seven days than the two experimental groups, each of which received one of the specific NSAIDs.[38]

Although you can do strength training effectively at home, when 74 Swedish women (age 57) with low back pain were randomly assigned either to back exercises at a fitness center and a home training program or to a home training program alone for 3 months, examination at 3 and 12 months, and a mailed questionnaire after three years, showed that while both groups manifested significant improvement, adherence rate was much better in the group assigned to the fitness center. Both groups continued to pursue the home training program after the first 3 months, and the home training program appeared as effective as the fitness center program after at least one year of adherence.[39]

Like aerobic exercise, strength training just makes you feel better and has also been shown to serve as an effective antidepressant in depressed elders. Thirty-two volunteers, ranging in age from 60 to 84 with major or minor depression, participated in a 10-week study that randomly assigned them to a supervised progressive strength program three times a week or a control group. No significant adverse effects occurred in the exercise group, while bodily pain, depression, quality of life, vitality, and social functioning significantly improved. Strength increased 33 percent in the exercisers and actually decreased 2 percent for the controls.[40]

FLEXIBILITY TRAINING

Flexibility training aims at improving the range of motion around a joint. As we age, our joints lose some of their flexibility, plus inactivity causes the connective tissue around the joints to shorten. Stretching can help prevent the shortening or tightening of muscles of the back and lower legs, and a supple body allows you to exercise aerobically with greater ease. It reduces the risk of injury to joints, muscles, and tendons. When done before and after aerobic exercise or strength training, stretching can reduce cramping, muscle soreness, and muscle tension.

With stretching, all of us can increase our flexibility. Some of the additional benefits of flexibility training include a reduction in the risk of future injury, improved relaxation, and stress reduction. One of the most popular methods of stretching is what experts call "static stretching," where you move into the stretch just until you feel tension in the muscle but not pain. You're easing into a position of mild tension. Then you *hold* the stretch for 10 to 30 seconds. *Absolutely no bouncing,* regardless of what you've been taught or all the old army movies you've seen where recruits in boot camp are led through their exercises with a "one-two-three" drill. When a muscle is rapidly jerked into extension (up-down, up-down), it contracts or tightens, a reaction called the "stretch reflex." The muscle utilizes it as a means of self-protection against overstretching. The muscle being "stretched" is, in fact, actually tightening, increasing the likelihood of injury.

It is important in stretching to breathe correctly. Exhaling as you stretch the muscle or hold the tension (exerting effort) helps regulate blood pressure. Breathe slowly through the nose, expanding the abdomen (not the chest). The rhythmic contraction and expansion of the abdominal blood helps to remove waste products from the muscles in the torso. Increased blood flow to the stretched muscles improves their elasticity and increases the rate at which lactic acid is purged from them.

Warmth increases the benefits of flexibility training, so choose a warm room, or wear warm clothing if you're stretching outside.

Yoga offers a series of good flexibility exercises, ones that you can participate in at your own pace, whatever your age and condition.

Experts suggest that you ought to add stretching to your fitness routine in 20- to 30-minute sessions three times a week in the beginning. Precede it by a 5- to 10-minute warm-up period in which you rhythmically move all your major muscle groups in order to send blood to the muscles.

As with all other fitness activities, increase the number of times and amount of time you engage in flexibility training *gradually*. Gentle, low-intensity stretching performed daily helps to maintain or improve range of motion and is the foundation of most therapeutic exercise programs. It is also important in recreational exercise or fitness programs. Adequate flexibility improves function and reduces the chance of injury during other activities.

Stretching doesn't require that you go to a gym or develop an intensive fitness program. It can be done any time of the day and almost anywhere. There are videocassettes to motivate and guide you, if you have trouble getting started.

EXERCISE TIPS

Pain and weakness often discourage chronically ill persons from being physically active, but the more primary obstacles are lack of motivation and lack of knowledge. Given an *individualized* exercise regimen that both motivates and instructs, people tend to exercise more frequently and more safely and to become aware of the benefit of exercise therapy as an adjuvant to their medical treatment.[41] Check with your doctor first, and then consider joining a gym or working with a personal trainer to get you started on a program that is right for you.

Warm-up routines before hard exercise are important in order to avoid stress injuries, such as muscle cramps, pains, and strains. Begin a walking or jogging program with some stretches and then walk slowly for several minutes, and jog slowly before getting up to speed. Warm-up exercises that do not use the same muscles you are going to be exercising are of little value in protecting you from the stress injuries of that exercise.

Likewise, cooling down after exercise by walking slowly or otherwise moving for about five minutes, rather than standing still, is extremely important. An estimated 65 percent of all severe heart problems occur as you stop activity.[42] Avoid standing still and never sit down immediately after vigorous activity. Continued movement to gradually bring your heart rate to normal can prevent arrhythmia that could follow because of the enormous amounts of blood vessel constrictor hormones (norepinephrine and epinephrine) that continue to be produced for several minutes after exercise stops.[43]

While it is true that exercise promotes muscle and bone

development, it is also true that overexercise can result in the breakdown of muscle tissue and a significant loss of muscle mass, especially if repeated for many days. The older a person is, the greater the possibility that this will occur, since tissue repair tends to slow down with age.[44] So don't be compulsive about exercising. Use your magnets to allow you to gradually move more easily.

Don't engage in strenuous exercise for three hours after any meal that is high in fat. When your blood is filled with fat from a recent meal, it cannot carry as much oxygen as the body needs in order to perform aerobically.[45] A leisurely or moderately brisk walk, however, is fine.

If you're just beginning to exercise, small doses are often better than extensive ones. Do you realize that if you take six 10-minute walks, you've walked for an hour, whereas if we told you that you had to walk an hour every day, you would probably think to yourself that we don't understand your pain. If part of your body hurts during those brief walks, strap or tape your magnets on. Then take a rest; you've earned it.

By the way, six little rest breaks scattered throughout the day are better for pain relief than one or two longer ones. Gradually as you build up your strength and endurance, you will be able to engage in longer, more sustained physical fitness activities.

This technique of spacing out your activities is called *pacing* and is very beneficial in relieving or controlling pain. Pacing allows you to break up your day by balancing and spacing rest or relaxation with activity.[46] Put simply, pacing involves doing many of your activities in short intervals of time. This requires you initially to be sensitive to how much time you can spend at a particular task before your pain increases, then stop the pain-increasing activities *before* your pain begins, thus achieving pain control.

Before you start any exercise program it is important to check with your doctor. If you are over 40, an exercise tolerance test may be ordered to rule out any cardiovascular problems that might require exercise restrictions. In all likelihood your doctor will applaud your resolve and help you set up an exercise plan. Joining a gym or working with a personal trainer, especially for the first few months, is another way to get started on the right track.

Whatever approach toward exercise you choose, strap on your magnets, and get moving!

Chapter Nine

NUTRITIONAL HEALING: YOU *FEEL* WHAT YOU EAT

Although there is no specific diet that will keep you pain free for the rest of your life, as a correlate to magnet therapy there *are* things you can do nutrition-wise to help you feel better and have less pain. There are specific foods that either promote or lessen the pain response, foods that make you feel worse or better.

The banana, for instance, provides, among other nutrients, the amino acid tryptophan, a precursor for serotonin, a neurotransmitter or chemical messenger in the brain that helps regulate mood (low levels of serotonin have been linked to depression). Eat a banana, feel better. Experiencing aches and pains of arthritis? Have some salmon. The fats in salmon have a dampening effect on the prostaglandins your body produces that cause inflammation.

Well, it's not quite that simple, but perhaps you begin to get the idea. Nutrients in the food you eat, absorbed through your gastrointestinal tract, allow your body to manufacture chemical messengers in your brain, as well as prostaglandins throughout your body, that have serious consequences in how you feel.[1]

Your body needs protein, which provides amino acids, the building blocks of muscles, enzymes, and other body tissues. It needs carbohydrates for energy, and fat to make hormones and healthy cell membranes. Other components the body needs from food are vitamins, the complex organic molecules required by all living organisms for healthy life and growth, and minerals: calcium, phosphorus, sodium, chloride, potassium, magnesium, and trace minerals.[2]

Beginning to understand why it's essential that you follow a healthful, varied diet? How else are you going to get the basic nutrients you need for optimal health — and to stimulate the production of neurotransmitters and other pain-relieving substances?

When we snack or eat, most of us think in terms of what we crave, what we like, what's in the kitchen, whether we are on a diet and what's allowed on the diet. Few of us think in terms of the meal providing us with "brain food" or specific components we need to feel better. How many times have you approached a meal saying or thinking, "Yum, I've got to feed my brain" or "I really need to monitor my prostaglandin production"? But in order to feel good and minimize pain, maybe you should.

It is not our intent in this chapter to get involved in discussing which diet might be the correct one for you, but rather to explain in general the important ingredients that should make up your daily diet and how they affect your body's functioning, especially with regard to pain and pain relief.

WHAT SHOULD I EAT?

Diet has been a big part of Dr. Whitaker's medical practice for over 25 years. He advocates a diet low in saturated fats and simple carbohydrates, such as refined flour and sweets, with larger amounts of vegetables and fruits (essential sources of fiber, vitamins, and minerals) and moderate lean protein sources.

The emphasis here is on plant foods, and we recommend a minimum of five — and preferably twice that — half-cup servings of fruit and vegetables daily. An easy way to make sure you get enough is to picture one serving as being the size of the palm of your hand or of a tennis ball. For raw leafy greens, however, one serving equals two palms or tennis balls.

This diet is a far cry from the one recommended for early Greek athletes by Diogenes Laertius, a writer who lived in the early decades of the third century. At that time, athletes trained on dried figs, moist cheese, and wheat.[3] Makes you happy to eat all those greens, doesn't it? If you have arthritis, you'll be even happier, since medical research has shown that a vegetarian diet can dramatically reduce arthritic pain.[4] If you don't want to become a vegetarian, just be sure to add more vegetables to your diet.

GET YOUR FILL OF PHYTOCHEMICALS

Although vegetables, fruits, legumes, and beans — plant foods — are the richest sources of vitamins and minerals in your diet, many of these nutrients can be derived from animal sources as well.

One component, however, is unique to plant foods, and that is *phytochemicals* (*phyto* meaning "plant"). Phytochemicals, which number in the tens of thousands, protect plants from the insults of their environment, and when eaten provide powerful health benefits for us as well.[5]

Some of the most potent phytochemicals are the carotenoids; the best known of these is beta-carotene, found in carrots and other yellow vegetables. Other carotenoids, lutein and zeaxanthin, are found in dark leafy greens and have been shown to reduce macular degeneration, the leading cause of blindness in elderly people. Lycopene, the carotenoid that makes tomatoes red, has been shown to protect men from prostate cancer.

Cruciferous vegetables, such as broccoli and cabbage, are a good source of indoles, which are protective against cancer.

Artichokes contain cymarin, an extract that promotes liver regeneration and acts as a protective compound against liver-damaging agents. Cayenne (red pepper), thyme, turmeric, rosemary, cumin, fennel, garlic, green tea, cloves, and cinnamon all have important antioxidant phytochemicals. Quercetin, found in onions, is a particularly powerful antioxidant that also has antihistamine effects. Blueberries, Concord grapes, and strawberries (which have one of the highest antioxidant capacities among the fruits and vegetables) are abundant sources of flavonoids. (See chapter 10 for a discussion of antioxidants and flavonoids.)

Soybeans (found in tofu, soy milk, soy meat substitutes, and Japanese miso soup) are a rich source of isoflavones, which are being studied for their tumor-suppressing effects. Soybeans also deliver a substance to the body called phosphatidylserine, which improves concentration, memory, and mood. It helps "brain cells conduct nerve impulses and enhances the release of neurotransmitters that carry messages from one cell to another."[6]

Remember: Although you can take vitamin supplements that contain beta-carotene and a few other phytochemicals, the full range of these intrinsic food factors can be obtained only by eating copious amounts of fruits and vegetables.

FUN WITH FIBER

Plant foods also provide us with fiber, which used to be called roughage. All dietary fiber comes from plants. Fibers are classified as insoluble and soluble, and we need both. Insoluble fiber (found in vegetables, especially celery, wheat and corn bran, and the skins of fruits and root vegetables) doesn't dissolve in water. It helps prevent gastrointestinal disorders and constipation. Soluble fiber, which forms a gel-like substance in water and is found in oats and oat bran, beans, peas, carrots, citrus fruits, and apples, can lower blood cholesterol, and slows the absorption of blood sugar, making sugar levels easier to control. This makes for more energy.

We recommend that you eat at least 30 grams of fiber a day (count 2 grams for each serving of whole-grain foods, fruits, or vegetables and 10 grams for each serving of beans). If you haven't been eating that much, increase your intake gradually — say an additional 5 grams every couple of weeks, allowing your body to adjust. Too much fiber too fast may lead to gas and a bloated feeling.

PROTEIN

We need amino acids, nitrogen-containing molecules, not only to aid in the production of neurotransmitters but to provide the building blocks for proteins, which make up most of your body's tissues. The body breaks down the proteins you eat into amino acids, then reassembles them into the essential proteins required for enzymes, hormones, muscle fibers, and other tissues.

The 9 essential amino acids, including tryptophan, the one in bananas, necessary to build protein for the body have to come from your diet, because the body can't manufacture them. The other 11 amino acids needed by the body can either be manufactured in your intestines and liver or obtained from your diet.

The best protein sources are low-fat, lean poultry, seafood, egg whites, and low-fat dairy products. Lentils, beans, and many grains — especially quinoa, amaranth, and teff, a tiny grain from Egypt — also have significant amounts of protein.

WHAT ABOUT FAT?

By now most of us have heard alarming descriptions of how fat, especially saturated fat, clogs the vessels that carry blood to the heart and also promotes brain deterioration by clogging the vessels that carry oxygen and glucose to the brain. Variation in the intake of saturated fat may explain why the incidence of coronary heart disease varies among different countries.[7]

How much fat is too much? There the authorities differ. Many think it is important to keep your intake of fat below 20 percent of your total calories.[8] Dr. Dean Ornish, the well-known developer of a holistic program for reversing heart disease and author of several books, does not even allow that much in his program. He restricts fat to less than 10 percent of your total calories. His vegetarian diet also prohibits caffeine and animal products except egg whites, nonfat milk, and yogurt.

By contrast, the famed Mediterranean diet, said by some to be one of the world's most healthful, allows 30 to 40 percent fat. In the diet of the Mediterranean countries of Greece and Italy, the main fat is olive oil, and its high consumption is considered a major contributor to the diet's disease-preventive aspects.

Researchers in France randomly placed 302 patients who had recently had a first heart attack (myocardial infarction) on the Mediterranean diet and compared their incidence of having a second attack with that of a control group of 303 patients who were placed on the standard therapeutic diet. After an average follow-up of 27 months, there were only 3 cardiac deaths and 5 nonfatal myocardial infarctions in the Mediterranean diet group versus 16 cardiac deaths and 17 nonfatal myocardial infarctions in the control group.[9]

We recommend the middle ground. At Dr. Whitaker's clinic in Newport Beach, California, where patients from all over the country come and stay for a week of medical evaluation and nutrition, exercise, and lifestyle instruction, the emphasis is on complex carbohydrates (60–70 percent), lean protein (15–20 percent), and healthy fats (15–20 percent). One way to achieve this healthy-fat ratio is by cutting down on beef and other saturated-fat sources and replacing them with the lower-fat protein sources mentioned above. And remember, the foundation of this healthy diet is plant foods, especially vegetables and fruits.

ESSENTIAL FATTY ACIDS: ESSENTIAL FOR HEALTH

The low-fat craze has missed the mark. The truth is that fat, consumed in moderate amounts, is important to the body. Fat slows the release of sugar into your bloodstream, helping to sustain energy. Fat is necessary for the absorption of vitamins A, E, D, and K, and beta-carotene, and for the formation of all cell membranes.

In fact, some fats are crucial to optimal health, so much so that they are termed *essential fatty acids* (EFAs). These are divided into two categories: linoleic acid, sometimes called omega-6 (found in nuts, seeds, vegetable oils, most grains, and beans), and alpha-linolenic acid, sometimes called omega-3 (found in flaxseed, salmon, and other cold-water fish). The omega-3 oils are especially important in pain prevention and control, as they have anti-inflammatory, pain-relieving properties.[10] It is difficult to get adequate omega-3 EFAs in your diet, and we recommend supplementing them, as detailed later in chapter 10.

TO FEEL BETTER, EAT LESS FAT

A number of studies have been conducted on the effects of fat on mood. A breakfast high in fat makes you feel less alert, vigorous, and imaginative, more "dreamy, feeble, and fatigued."[11] After feeding them breakfasts that varied in fat and carbohydrate composition, researchers asked a group of persons to carry out a series of computer-based cognitive tasks that had been shown to be sensitive to dietary effects. Although various food combinations didn't seem to make a difference in performance, they did have significant effects on mood.

Mood improved following a low-fat, high-carbohydrate meal. The effects were independent of meal size and of any obvious differences in the sensory quality of the breakfasts.[12]

It appears that mood is related to higher concentrations of plasma insulin after low-fat, high-carbohydrate meals, while high-fat, low-carbohydrate meals increase the production of cholecystokinin, which apparently increases feelings of lassitude.[13]

Insomnia is connected with low levels of the neurotransmitter serotonin, a condition that is linked to a variety of emotional disorders and stress-related complaints. Most of the newer antidepressant medications (Prozac, Zoloft) boost existing serotonin by delaying its absorption. Ineffective when administered orally as a supplement, serotonin can be enhanced by increasing the intake of its precursor, tryptophan.* Pasta, turkey, fresh green beans, eggplant, apricots, cherries, pears, and pumpkin seeds are all foods high in natural tryptophan. Interestingly, depressed persons feel better after a low-fat, high-carbohydrate meal, as they boost their tryptophan/serotonin levels.

---

*In the 1980s, the FDA took tryptophan supplements off the shelves of health food stores after contaminants (not the tryptophan itself) in a batch from one Japanese manufacturer caused an outbreak of a sometimes deadly inflammatory disorder called eosinophilia myalgia syndrome (EMS). Although the problem was immediately identified and rectified, the ban on tryptophan inexplicably stayed in place for years — despite the fact that the amino acid continued to be added to baby formulas and IV preparations. Tryptophan is once again available, but only on a prescription basis, and it is perfectly safe. Since tryptophan is an amino acid naturally occurring in some foods and in the body, brain levels may also be increased by eating tryptophan-rich foods.

CARBOHYDRATES: SIMPLE OR COMPLEX?

The basic fuel of the body is glucose, which is derived from carbohydrates. (*Blood sugar* and *blood glucose* refer to the same thing.) Glucose is soluble in blood and cell fluids and available to all tissues for their energy needs.[14] Dr. Arthur Winter, a neurosurgeon, estimates that the brain alone consumes "a whopping 50 percent" of the body's glucose.[15]

Carbohydrates are simply foods rich in sugars that your body can break down into glucose. How those sugars are arranged determines whether we call them simple or complex carbohydrates. Fruit juice, white sugar, honey, maple syrup, white flour, and white rice are considered simple carbohydrates because the body can easily digest the tiny single or twin molecules they contain and get glucose into the bloodstream quickly. A meal heavy on simple carbohydrates will give you a quick, sharp increase in blood sugar, but it may drop just as rapidly, leaving you irritable and without energy. Although fruits contain the simple sugar fructose, it is bound up with fiber, thus slowing down its release into the bloodstream. Always choose whole fruit over fruit juice. Not only are you throwing away valuable fiber when you drink juice, but a tall glass of juice contains almost as much sugar as you'd get in a soda!

Complex carbohydrates (vegetables, whole grains, beans, lentils) are digested slowly and release a steady flow of glucose. They consist of groups of simple sugars bound together in long molecular chains that take the body longer to break down into glucose, providing energy over a longer period. Some carbohydrates are recombined to form glycogen, which is stored in the liver and muscles as a reserve energy source. Moderate or intense athletic activity will soon deplete your muscles' glycogen stores. This is the reason that athletes who rest for several days before a competition, while at the same time loading up on carbohydrates, have more stored glycogen, hence more endurance.

A DRINK OF COOL, CLEAR WATER

All too often, people in pain, especially those with an accompanying depression, neglect to eat or to drink fluids, which can cause or escalate health problems. We remember a science fiction show in which aliens from outer space looked at humans and decided they were "ugly bags of water." We didn't think the aliens were so beautiful either, but it is true that our bodies are about 60 percent water. The leaner a person is, the greater his or her percentage of water, since muscle cells contain more water than fat cells do.

Water has many functions; therefore, we require quite a lot of it. In emergencies, we can last much longer without food than without water. In general, we need a minimum of 8 glasses (64 ounces) a day to maintain our fluid balance, and 10 to 12 is even better. Water controls the body's temperature and carries nutrients and gases around the body. It assists in metabolizing stored fat and reducing fat deposits. Sufficient water helps reduce sodium (salt) buildup and helps the kidneys rid the body of waste and toxins. When your kidneys don't get enough water, your liver, which metabolizes fat, has to help the kidneys and can't fully do its own job.

Water also plays an important role in musculoskeletal pain. Many of us, unbeknownst to ourselves, are chronically dehydrated. We just don't drink enough water. Considering that over 50 percent of the cartilage in your joints and discs is made of water, it is easy to see how dehydration would contribute to osteoarthritis, which involves degenerative changes and wearing away of the cartilage.

Exercise, stress, dieting, and certain diseases increase the body's need for water. So keep that "fountain of life" coming.

IT DON'T MEAN A THING IF IT AIN'T GOT THAT ZING

Caffeine, the chemical most of us think we can't live without, is one of the world's most widely used drugs. Legend says that we have an Ethiopian goat herder to thank for our obsession with coffee. It was he who observed that his goats stayed awake all night when they nibbled on the berries of the *Coffea arabica* bush. He tried the berries himself and passed along the practice.[16]

Caffeine stimulates all parts of the central nervous system, causing vasoconstriction. It is a xanthine, and what xanthines do generally is increase your heart rate and raise your blood sugar. That's the lift or surge of energy you feel after drinking a cup of coffee. Too soon, however, your body reacts by reducing the amount of sugar in your blood, causing fatigue, hunger, and, psychologically, the need to pour yourself another cup of coffee. Since caffeine promotes diuresis, the increased excretion of urine, too much caffeine also leads to dehydration.

A cup of coffee in the morning is probably fine, but high intakes of caffeine may have many detrimental health effects. Excess caffeine can decrease bone mineral mass by causing reduced absorption of and increased urinary excretion of calcium, which means a greater chance of developing osteoporosis.[17] It also promotes excretion of thiamine and other B vitamins, and can reduce the absorption of iron.[18] Caffeine may cause restlessness, insomnia, ringing in the ears (tinnitus), anxiety, irritability, heartburn, digestive problems, diarrhea, rapid heartbeat (tachycardia), and even irregular heartbeat (arrhythmia).

When high-frequency, low-intensity TENS was used in a double-blind study to test the intensity and unpleasantness of thermally induced pain on the forearm of men in their twenties, it was found that following the administration of a placebo (no caffeine), TENS significantly reduced the intensity of heat-pain perception. After 200 mg of caffeine, however, TENS had no effect on either the perceived intensity or the perceived unpleasantness of painful heat.[19] It is possible, then, that caffeine may affect pain perception.

A number of over-the-counter pain relievers contain caffeine. There is some controversy over the rationale for its presence and whether or not the included caffeine enhances the effectiveness of the analgesics. Some believe it does. By reducing the dosage of the analgesic required to relieve pain, it may reduce the dose-related risks associated with the product's use.[20] Others say there is not enough caffeine in the products to make a difference. One doctor argues that the concentrations found in mild analgesics are less than half of what you could obtain by drinking a cup of coffee with an analgesic that has no caffeine.[21] After continued use of caffeinated medications, however, persons who stop taking them may develop a rebound headache that can last from one to five days, likely as rebound vasodilation of blood vessels in or to the head.[22] Headache is also one of the most prominent symptoms of caffeine withdrawal in general, and the only one to extend into the third day of withdrawal.[23]

The consumption of caffeine slows the absorption of oral medication, so persons with migraine headaches who take in large amounts of caffeine may experience a worsening of their headache, possibly promoting excessive analgesic use. An increase in caffeine use can also cause more headaches for persons who suffer the muscle-contraction variety, especially if they drink more coffee at the same time they increase their use of medications containing caffeine.

If you have insomnia or difficulty going to sleep at night, pay attention to the times at which you drink a beverage with caffeine (coffee, cola, chocolate milk, hot chocolate, tea) and determine whether or not it affects your pain or sleep level.

Sensitivity to caffeine may increase during pregnancy and as you grow older. If you have high blood pressure, gastritis, or ulcers, caffeine consumption can aggravate your condition.

Drip coffee has the highest amount of caffeine (around 120–150 mg per cup), with percolated (80–110 mg) falling not far behind and instant (60–70 mg) scoring third. Decaffeinated coffee has the least, of course, but still can contain as much as 3 to 10 mg per cup. Black tea has about half the amount of caffeine as drip coffee (50–60 mg), while green tea has 30–40 mg of caffeine. Most herbal teas don't contain caffeine. Cocoa and chocolate milk can range from 10 to 30 mg.

Our favorite pick-me-up in the mornings is green tea. It contains one-third to half the caffeine of coffee, yet it has enough to give you a heightened sense of alertness. In addition, green tea contains polyphenols, which have antioxidant, antibacterial, cholesterol-lowering, and tumor-suppressing properties. Give it a try. You may find that it wakes you up but doesn't leave you with that jagged feeling coffee sometimes does.

THE DOUBTFUL DUO: ALCOHOL AND CIGARETTES

Sometimes people turn to alcohol to control pain. Although it may take the edge off your pain initially, you're probably going to end up feeling worse, as alcohol is a depressant. The medical research shows that moderate drinking (one or two drinks a day) does confer a protective effect on the heart, but any more than that increases the risk of heart disease, cancer, and premature death.

Some people use alcohol as a sleep aid, but it doesn't really work well for this, either. While it may make you feel more relaxed at the time you drink it, it can cause you to awaken during the night and have difficulty falling asleep again. This is because the alcohol has depressed your blood sugar level, and one of the consequences of low blood sugar is insomnia.

In addition to adding useless calories to your diet and possibly increasing your weight — a problem for persons with pain in the lower part of their body — alcohol also interferes with the body's production of endorphins. Alcohol and cigarette smoke are two well-known triggers of cluster headaches, a periodic and particularly difficult type of headache to treat.

We have nothing positive to say about smoking. In addition to the fact that it dramatically increases your risk for heart disease, cancer, and just about any other degenerative disease you can think of, cigarette smoking is also associated with depressive symptoms.[24]

Several research studies also show that smokers experience more intense pain than nonsmokers, especially persons younger than 67.[25] In a British study of more than 34,000 persons, obesity and smoking were associated with back pain in both sexes and all ages, from 18 to 65 and beyond.[26] A 12-year follow-up study carried out in Finland to evaluate the risk factors for unspecified low back pain and sciatic pain indicated a close association between smoking and the prevalence of sciatic pain and suggested that smoking is a causal risk factor for lumbar disc disease.[27]

"DECEITFUL SWEET DAINTIES"

While many of us can pass up Aunt Fanny's Christmas fruitcake with ease, during the rest of the year we indulge in plenty of those "deceitful sweet dainties." In fact, according to the U.S. Department of Agriculture, on the average every American eats a staggering 149 pounds of sugar a year.

Our taste for sweets is innate. Even newborn babies will suck more vigorously on a bottle filled with sweetened water. This preference for sweets may have once helped steer us away from poisonous, bitter foods and toward the sweeter, safe ones.[28] However, excess sugar has a definite dark side. It wreaks havoc with blood glucose levels, causes dental cavities, and depletes the body of certain vitamins and minerals. In addition, sugar weakens the immune system by slowing down the motility of white blood cells and inhibiting the production of several disease-fighting hormones for as long as five hours after eating it, making us more prone to illness and pain.

AVOID POSSIBLE ALLERGENS

The body's responses to a food it cannot tolerate are varied. You might get a headache, increased mucus, sinus drainage, anxiety, depression, bloating, abdominal pain, diarrhea, aches and pains throughout the body . . . in other words, allergens may trigger a broad range of reactions, and pain is one of them.

It is estimated that over half of us have some kind of food sensitivities or allergies. They can be to anything, but the most common reactions are to dairy products, gluten (found in wheat, oats, barley, and rye), corn, sugar, and for arthritis pain, some claim, members of the nightshade family: tomatoes, peppers, potatoes, eggplant, and tobacco. Sometimes simply by identifying and removing from your diet an offending food, you will alleviate or even eliminate your headaches and other miscellaneous aches and pains.

In a 1991 study published in *The Lancet,* 27 patients with rheumatoid arthritis were enrolled for four weeks at a health spa. They first fasted for 7 to 10 days, then foods were gradually introduced back into their diets. They were monitored for increases in pain, stiffness, or swelling, and if any of these symptoms occurred within 48 hours of eating the food, the food was left out for a week. If they had a second reaction with the same food, it was completely eliminated from their diet.

They were then asked to continue on these custom diets, and during the study period to eat no meat, fish, eggs, dairy products, gluten-containing grains, sugar, citrus, salt, strong spices, alcohol, tea, or coffee. After 13 months, the patients on the restricted diet were compared to another group on a regular diet, and the former group had significant reduction in pain and stiffness, as well as objective decreases in swelling and joint tenderness, and increases in grip strength.[29]

The easiest way to confirm a suspected food intolerance is to eliminate that food from your diet for a couple of weeks and then reintroduce it, noting changes in symptoms.

HEADACHE-CAUSING FOODS

It has been known for some time that certain foods, additives, and other substances will trigger several types of headaches, particularly migraines. In some cases dietary changes can completely stop migraine headaches. In others they only reduce the frequency of attacks. Foods containing sodium nitrate, nitrites, monosodium glutamate (MSG), tyramine (chocolate, aged cheese, red wine), and aspartame have also been implicated in causing headaches.[30] Tyramine acts on sympathetic-nerve fibers, releasing norepinephrine and adrenaline and causing vasoconstriction similar to the "fight or flight" response. The headache that follows likely results from a rebound vasodilation.[31]

Other foods known to provoke migraine headaches are coffee, alcohol, yogurt, bananas, dried fruit, beans, pickled and marinated foods, and buttermilk.

Chapter Ten

TO SUPPLEMENT
OR NOT TO SUPPLEMENT

A myth widely circulated in the medical community holds that we can get all the vitamins, minerals, and other nutrients we need simply by eating right. But who eats right? And even if you do, are you sure that the food you're eating contains all the nutrients you need?

It is just plain naive to assume that you can get optimal nutrition through diet alone. Poor eating habits, inferior soil quality, prolonged storing and processing of food — plus the additional nutritional needs that the stressors of modern life create for us all — virtually assure that we're not getting all the vitamins and minerals we need through our food.

Tens of thousands of clinical studies have demonstrated the value of various nutritional supplements, not only to prevent or slow down degenerative diseases but to improve vitality, energy, and mood, and even to provide pain relief. But don't count on your doctor to recommend nutritional supplements. Most just choose to ignore the evidence — or perversely suppress it. Here's an interesting example of what we mean.

Jason Mehta, a ninth-grade student in Gainesville, Florida, surveyed 181 cardiologists who themselves had coronary artery disease. Almost half (44 percent) reported taking antioxidant supplements, which we will discuss below, for their potential benefits, with vitamin E being the most prevalent (39 percent). Vitamin C followed a close second (33 percent), while 19 percent of the doctors took beta-carotene. Yet only 37 percent of these doctors routinely recommended antioxidants to their patients with heart disease.

Dr. Whitaker is considered an expert in the field of nutritional supplementation, as he has been using it, along with diet, exercise, and other lifestyle changes, with his patients for over 20 years, often with astounding results. Here is a brief explanation of one of the most important classes of supplements, antioxidants, as well as his general recommendations for nutritional supplementation.

FREE RADICALS AND ANTIOXIDANTS

If "free radicals" sounds like a political group bent on insurrection, you're not far from wrong, only the insurrection is in our own bodies. Most of the characteristics of aging, including cataracts, gray hair, wrinkled skin, memory loss, and many diseases, including arthritis, cancer, and heart disease, result from the cellular damage caused by free radicals, extremely reactive, unstable molecules released during the course of normal metabolic activities that consume oxygen.

Under normal circumstances, molecules and their building blocks, atoms, retain a certain stability; however, when an atom or molecule loses one of its paired electrons through normal metabolic processes, such as breathing or extracting energy from food, or from pollution or ultraviolet radiation, what is left is a free radical.

Highly reactive, free radicals steal electrons from other molecules they come in contact with, causing them to become unstable as well. Free radicals injure cell membranes, cause inflammation, induce mutations in DNA and genes, and cause widespread and bizarre disturbances in normal cellular function. Damage from free radicals is called oxidation, and there's no way to avoid it.

Your body has numerous mechanisms to carefully control and coordinate free-radical activity. Their destructive action is normally neutralized by natural antioxidants made in the body, which scavenge the body to seek out the free radicals and render them harmless. In addition, foods and supplements high in antioxidants can help keep the insurrection in check.

Increased exposure to cigarette smoke, air pollution, sunlight, radiation, pesticides, polyunsaturated fats, and stress all generate increased amounts of free radicals. Overexercising, excessive drinking, overeating, weight loss, sleep deprivation, infections, impaired liver or kidney function, genetic factors, and even the altitude at which you live (high altitudes cause more free radicals to be produced due to higher levels of exposure to atmospheric radiation) also affect antioxidant requirements due to the production of free radicals.

The bad news is that our ability to manufacture antioxidants declines under conditions of increased stress, and as we grow older. The good news is that antioxidant vitamins, minerals, herbal extracts, and combinations of these can help block the damage caused by free radicals.

VITAMIN VITALITY

Let's take a moment to review the importance of the various vitamins for the body, particularly with respect to their effect on pain, depression, and stress. Please note that each vitamin has many other important functions as well.

Vitamins can be classed as water-soluble (vitamin C and the vitamins in the B-complex) because they dissolve readily in water, and fat-soluble (vitamins A, D, E, K, and beta-carotene), which dissolve more readily in oil.

Vitamin A comes in two forms. As vitamin A, it is found in liver, eggs, butter, cod liver oil, and fortified dairy products. As **beta-carotene** it is the phytochemical responsible for the color of carrots, sweet potatoes, red peppers, winter squash, apricots, cantaloupes, mangoes, and peaches.

Vitamin A is necessary for maintaining good vision, the growth of bone and glands, the inner linings of the body (mucous membranes), cell membranes, and a healthily functioning immune system. A vitamin A deficiency can affect how iron is used by your body. It is depleted by alcohol, cortisone (used to treat inflammation), and by intestinal, kidney, or liver diseases. The recommended supplemental dose of vitamin A is 5,000 IU daily; of beta-carotene, 15,000 IU (and many of these recommendations are much higher than the RDAs).

Among their many other functions, the **B-complex vitamins** help us maintain a strong immune system. They are involved in energy production, which makes them essential for persons with low energy levels and fatigue, and those with chronic fatigue syndrome. B-complex vitamins also help support the adrenal glands, one of the major organs connected with stress. When faced with danger, for example, the adrenal glands pump out the hormone adrenaline. The result is a faster pulse, an increase in blood pressure, and heightened awareness — commonly known as the "fight or flight" response. They have also been found helpful in treating peripheral neuralgia (pain in a nerve of the arms, legs, shoulders, neck, or scalp).

They are depleted by stress, environmental pollution, and the ingestion of sugar, white flour, and alcohol.

B1, or **thiamine** (found in whole grains, meats, fish, poultry, legumes, nuts, and seeds), is needed for the breakdown of food into energy; hence, deficiencies of it can lead to fatigue, irritability, sleep disturbance, and chest pain. People who frequently use aspirin or antacids risk developing a thiamine deficiency. Severe deficiencies can result in numbness, calf muscle cramps, and leg pains. You should supplement with 50 mg per day.

B2 (riboflavin) helps the body produce red blood cells, and activates a powerful antioxidant, glutathione, to fight toxic chemicals and free radicals. Its main sources are milk and liver, although other good sources are sunflower seeds, broccoli, butternut squash, wild rice, brown rice, and almonds. Without riboflavin the body is unable to use B6. Some tranquilizers and tricyclic antidepressants deplete riboflavin or inhibit its breakdown. The recommended supplement is 50 mg per day.

Excellent sources of **B3 (niacin** or **niacinamide)** include meat, poultry, dairy products, tuna, tofu, nuts, and seeds. Niacin is made in the intestines from the amino acid tryptophan, and is known to lower cholesterol and aid in the reduction of osteoarthritic inflammation. It can also counteract some of the effects of caffeine. B3 deficiency can cause anxiety, fatigue, depression, and loss of short-term memory. An adequate daily dose of vitamin B3 is 20 mg, although its therapeutic dose may be significantly increased to combat high cholesterol.

Pantothenic acid, also known as **B5,** is necessary for optimal energy levels, for wound healing, and for maintaining a strong immune system. It is important to persons under stress, in order to allow the adrenal glands to manufacture their hormones and in order to maintain their ability to produce such hormones after depletion. The adrenals also help convert fat and glucose into energy.

Sleeping pills, alcohol, caffeine, and estrogen destroy pantothenic acid. Good sources are eggs, milk, fresh vegetables, and bran. You need 50 mg of B5 daily.

B6 (pyridoxine) is necessary for brain function, the growth of red blood cells, immune system functioning, and for the prevention and treatment of a wide range of degenerative diseases. Since B6 is needed for the production of the neurotransmitter serotonin, a deficiency can result in depression and mental confusion. It is important for metabolizing proteins, but too much protein leads to increased excretion of B6.

Vitamin B6 has also been shown to change pain thresholds in clinical and laboratory studies, which may be the reason it is able to reduce the pain of carpal tunnel syndrome. The carpal tunnel, a sheath of bones and tendons in your wrist, normally protects the median nerve, a major nerve to your hand. If the tunnel collapses and begins to squeeze the nerve, the result is carpal tunnel syndrome, a debilitating and painful condition. Compression of the nerve in the arm or shoulder can also cause carpal tunnel pain. When 20 adults with carpal tunnel syndrome ingested 200 mg of B6 a day for three months, they all showed significant decrease in pain.[1] Good sources of B6 are bananas, chicken, fish, eggs, oats, soybeans, tomatoes, salmon, kale, kidney beans, peanuts, and walnuts. An adequate daily dose for healthy individuals is 75 mg.

B12 is a crucial nutrient for a healthy nervous system, helping the growth and maintenance of the myelin sheath (tissue that encases and protects the nerve fibers), and the development of red blood cells. B12 deficiency has been linked to paranoia, restlessness, irritability, chronic fatigue syndrome, memory loss, and insomnia. Since B12 is found only in animal (lean meat, fish) and dairy (milk, cottage cheese, yogurt) products, it is especially important for strict vegetarians to supplement their diet with it, as deficiencies can cause progressive and irreversible nerve damage. B12 is affected by aging, as the aging stomach may no longer secrete enough acid to separate B12 from protein. Deficiencies can also cause a loss of balance, numbness or weakness of the limbs, irritability, and mild depression. Alcohol, estrogen, and sleeping pills lower B12 levels. Recommended supplemental doses are 100 mcg per day, and more for people over 65.

Folic acid, a B-complex vitamin, helps in the division and replacement of red blood cells. It is needed for protein metabolism and the utilization of glucose. Deficiencies can cause irritability and gastrointestinal upsets, as well as neural tube birth defects and arteriosclerosis. Alcohol reduces the ability of the body to absorb it; aspirin and sunlight deplete it. Good sources are dark green leafy vegetables, carrots, apricots, beans (especially soy and navy beans), chicken liver, and walnuts. Some foods, such as orange juice, are fortified with folate, but it is not as well absorbed as supplemental folic acid. The recommended daily dose is 400 mcg.

Vitamin C (ascorbic acid) is a superb antioxidant that is synthesized by most animal species *except* humans. Circulating through the bloodstream and in body fluids, it neutralizes free radicals. When adequate vitamin C is present, the body can increase its production of lymphocyte T-cells and B-cells, major infection fighters. Vitamin C also protects against atherosclerosis and may play a role in cancer prevention.

While there are no studies that indicate vitamin C will prevent the development of arthritis, high levels of vitamin C have been shown to inhibit the progression of osteoarthritis of the knee. Good dietary sources of vitamin C are citrus fruits, strawberries, cantaloupe, watermelon, honeydew melon, red peppers, broccoli, brussels sprouts, and cauliflower. The recommended supplement is 2,500 mg per day.

Vitamin D, known as the "sunshine vitamin" because the body makes it after exposure to the sun, helps the body absorb calcium and ensures that there is enough in the blood for adequate bone formation. It has been shown to reduce the risk of osteoarthritis progression. Many foods, especially milk, are now supplemented with vitamin D, and natural nutritional sources include eggs, butter, cheese, and fish oil from sardines, salmon, and tuna.

This fat-soluble vitamin is readily stored in the body and excess is harmful. Prolonged excesses calcify tissues, accelerate aging, and cause heart disease and kidney damage.[2] A safe supplemental dose is 400 IU.

Vitamin E, found in peanut butter, almonds, filberts, sunflower seeds, shrimp, and vegetable oils, is a potent antioxidant. Cells with plenty of vitamin E in their membranes can resist the oxidative reactions of free radicals. It boosts synthesis of antibodies and encourages reproduction of lymphocytes, key infection-fighting cells. It has also been shown to keep inflammation and arthritis pain down by reducing the formation of prostaglandin E2, and to prevent the transformation of nitrite food additives into cancer-causing nitrosamine. Vitamin E, a potent antioxidant, stabilizes the membranes that insulate nerve fibers so they can carry their messages efficiently.[3] Studies show that taking supplemental vitamin E significantly reduces the risk of heart disease. Dr. Whitaker recommends supplementing with 800 IU a day.

MINERALS

Calcium, an important nutrient in pain relief, and especially good for painful leg cramps, is supplied in milk products. Calcium works synergistically with vitamin D, phosphorus, and magnesium. Yet too much phosphorus can interfere with calcium production, and specific proteins in dairy products can also deplete the body's supply of calcium.[4] Therefore, it is important to get extra calcium from vegetables like broccoli, cabbage, sea greens, and leafy greens, as well as nuts, seeds, and tofu. Calcium should be consumed in a ratio of 2 calcium to 1 phosphorus,[5] and the same ratio for magnesium.[6] Too much fat, oxalic acid (found in spinach, rhubarb, and chocolate), and phytic acid, found in grains, can also result in calcium deficiency.[7]

Calcium nourishes and calms the nervous system and is one of the most important nutrients for preventing bone loss. For people with osteoporosis, calcium, along with other nutrients, hormones, and weight-bearing exercise, can help prevent further deterioration of bones. Unfortunately, calcium is excreted when we consume excess protein or large amounts of sodas, which contain phosphoric acid.

Calcium supplements need to be taken with food for maximal effectiveness. There is some evidence that during the night, bone loss leaps 11 percent over daytime rates; therefore, bedtime may be the best time for taking a calcium supplement or calcium-rich snack.

Although milk has a number of nutritional and health benefits — a major one being protection against osteoporosis — contrary to popular belief, a glass of warm milk at bedtime does not bring on sleep, according to Jean Carper, author of *The Food Pharmacy*. Apparently the tiny amount of tryptophan (one-tenth of a gram per glass) in milk is rendered ineffective by the more plentiful amino acids in milk. In fact, as little as a half cup of skim milk or low-fat milk will actually stir up your mental energy, by delivering tyrosine to the brain, which in turn triggers production of dopamine and norepinephrine (neurotransmitters that stimulate the brain).[8]

You're better off with calcium supplements, 1,000 mg daily; 1,500 for those at risk for osteoporosis.

Magnesium is the mineral that Americans are most deficient in. Magnesium plays a number of important roles in the body. It normalizes heart rhythm, helps build healthy bones, increases muscle size in response to weight training, relieves muscle cramps, balances blood sugar (thereby sustaining energy), conducts nerve impulses, enhances the immune system, and protects the body from stress. Magnesium deficiency can be expressed as depression or agitation, confusion, and irritability. You'll find magnesium in nuts, seeds, tofu, oatmeal, whole grains, seafood, and leafy greens.

The German neurologist Andreas Peikert has discovered that magnesium effectively fights migraine headache, reducing the number of migraines in 56 percent of the group that received magnesium over a 16-week period compared to 31 percent for the placebo group.[9] Magnesium is also helpful in warding off leg cramps. The recommended daily dose of magnesium is 500 mg.

Potassium, found in all fruits, vegetables, nuts, and grains and particularly abundant in bananas, works to maintain the correct sodium balance in the body. It helps contract muscles, send messages between the nerves, and aids circulation, in part by dilating blood vessels. It is critical for maintaining optimal energy levels, so low levels of potassium deficiency may cause you to feel lethargic and weak. Most of your potassium needs are met through a healthy diet. Supplementing with 99 mg a day is also a good idea.

Iron is necessary to make red blood cells, which supply the body with oxygen. Our intake of iron has to be watched very carefully because it is easy to get too much, especially with so many iron-fortified foods on the market (cereals, white flour, and white rice, and products made from them). Couple those foods with a multivitamin tablet that has iron and it's easy to acquire an excess, which can create free radicals, increase the risk of heart disease, and feed pathogens that cause gastrointestinal infections. Good food sources of iron are animal products (meat, fish, poultry, and eggs), legumes, and dried fruits, which contain iron because they are dried in iron containers.[10]

Dr. Whitaker does not recommend that most people take supplemental iron. However, if you need extra iron, take your supplement with orange juice (the vitamin C makes it easier to absorb from supplements), and choose a ferrous, not ferric, compound, again because it is easier to absorb and causes less gastrointestinal irritation. A meal that includes foods high in iron should also include vitamin C–rich foods and fruits.[11]

Zinc is present in all organs and is vital to the activity of more than 100 enzymes.[12] It is quickly depleted by stress, and a deficiency will make it hard to keep the blood sugar level balanced or to digest food well. Zinc improves immune response, and helps the body utilize vitamin A. Megadoses inhibit calcium absorption when dietary calcium is low, while large amounts of iron in the diet can reduce the absorption of zinc. Chicken, turkey, shellfish (especially oysters), and pumpkin seeds are good sources of zinc. A good daily dose of zinc is 30 mg.

Copper plays an important role in boosting the immune system by making sure your T-cells and antibodies are armed and ready. Good sources of copper are shellfish, nuts, sesame seeds, mushrooms, and whole-grain cereals. Supplement in the range of 2 mg a day.

Chromium is a trace mineral found in brewer's yeast, wheat germ, whole wheat and rye bread, and potatoes. It helps control blood sugar levels, elevated triglycerides, cholesterol, and, when combined with other measures, weight. Chromium is the mineral most often depleted by excess sugar intake. The most easily absorbed form of this mineral is chromium picolinate, and a daily dose of 200 mcg is recommended.

Another trace mineral, **selenium,** has shown promise in recent years as a cancer preventive. In fact, a 1996 study was stopped before its completion once it was discovered that the people taking the mineral had such superior cancer protection — the researchers thought it unethical to withhold selenium from the control group. Dietary sources of selenium include wheat germ, Brazil nuts, oats, bran, barley, and whole wheat bread. Supplement recommendation is 200 mcg daily.

ESSENTIAL FATTY ACIDS

In chapter 9 we mentioned the importance of getting essential fatty acids (EFAs) in your diet. If you are suffering pain, you should take this one step further and actually supplement with omega-3 EFAs. Specifically, a component of omega-3, eicosopentaenoic acid (EPA), works on a similar, but more selective, pain-relieving principle as aspirin and other NSAIDs: it shuts down the production of pain- and inflammation-causing prostaglandins. It does this by inhibiting the production of the enzyme delta 5 desaturase, which is involved in the production of the E2 prostaglandins that cause inflammation and pain. It is also the precursor for another class of prostaglandins, E3, that also have anti-inflammatory activity.

In a double-blind, placebo-controlled study, three groups of 23 arthritic patients were followed for 12 months. The first group took six 1-gram capsules of olive oil every day, the second took six 1-gram capsules of fish oil, and the third took three 1-gram capsules of each of the two types of oil. All three groups noted improvements, but the best results were achieved by those who took six fish oil capsules every day.[13]

EPA in the form of two fish oil capsules a day (a 1,000-mg capsule contains 180 mg EPA) is recommended. This dose can be doubled, or even tripled, for further pain relief, if inflammation is at issue. Another good source of omega-3 EFAs is a quarter cup freshly ground flaxseeds, or one to two tablespoons flaxseed oil.

GET IT FROM THE HERB GARDEN

In Greek mythology, Asclepius, the god of healing, became so skilled in the use of plants that he could even restore the dead to life, and indeed every early civilization practiced some form of herbal medicine. Some of them, particularly those of China and India, had extremely complex and effective herbal remedies, many of which have stayed in use to this day. In fact, herbs remain the primary form of medicine for 80 percent of the world's population.

Even though herbs have long been out of favor with modern traditional physicians, many of our most useful drugs have their origins in the early medical folklore of plants. Some of these include reserpine (a tranquilizer and blood pressure medicine) from Indian snakeroot (*Rauvolfia serpentina*), digitoxin (for congestive heart failure) from foxglove (*Digitalis purpurea*), quinine (an antimalarial) from Peruvian bark (genus *Cinchona*), cocaine (a painkiller) from coca leaves (*Erythroxylon coca*), atropine (an anticholinergic) from deadly nightshade (*Atropa belladonna*), and, as we noted in chapter 6, morphine (another painkiller) from the opium poppy (*Papaver somniferum*). The main active ingredient in approximately 25 percent of all prescription drugs sold in the United States is derived from plants.[14]

Herbal medicine is making a comeback in this country. In 1993, Americans spent an estimated $1.5 billion on herbal remedies.[15] In 1996, Americans spent nearly $6 billion on nutritional supplements (everything from herbs to vitamins and minerals to enzymes), and the market is growing by 20 percent every year.[16]

There are hundreds, if not thousands, of individual herbs and herbal combinations in use somewhere on the planet. And many of them are used for pain relief. Although this list is by no means exhaustive, we want to highlight a few of the commonly available herbs and botanical medicines that are most efficacious in pain relief.

GREEN DRINKS

Green drinks are freeze-dried juice from the young shoots of wheat or barley grass. They contain an abundance of vitamins, minerals, and chlorophyll, with large concentrations of antioxidants and protective enzymes. This specific combination of nutrients provides remarkable relief from pain and inflammation in some people. The recommended dose is one to two teaspoons in water first thing in the morning on an empty stomach, and again later in the day. Green drinks have a grassy taste that takes some getting used to, but they can be a powerful tool in your pain relief arsenal.

BROMELAIN

Bromelain, an enzyme from pineapple, has special properties when taken on an empty stomach. Like aspirin and omega-3 EFAs, it suppresses prostaglandins and kinins, amino acids that, like prostaglandins, increase inflammation and pain. Bromelain therefore attacks pain and inflammation in two ways, and it is exceptionally effective in arthritic pain. Bromelain has an interesting effect on other medicines or medicinal herbs taken at the same time: it increases their efficacy. In addition, it helps the healing of wounds and reduces recovery time.[17] Bromelain must be taken on an empty stomach. Otherwise, it will act like a digestive enzyme and use up all its energy breaking down your food. Bromelain is measured in milk-clotting units (mcu/gram). I recommend taking 2,000 to 6,000 mcu daily between meals. Do not take this supplement if you have an allergy to pineapple.

BOSWELLA

Boswella, from the *Boswellia serrata* tree, has been used for centuries in Ayurvedic medicine (originating in India) for treating the pain of arthritis and other inflammatory conditions. In one study, carried out at the Government Medical College in Jammu, India, 175 patients with rheumatoid arthritis so severe they couldn't work (many were even bedridden) were given 400 mg of boswella daily. After eight weeks, 14 percent had excellent improvement in pain, 44 percent reported good response, and 30 percent had fair improvement.[18]

For inflammation-related pain, try 400 mg daily of boswella, taken in divided doses.

TURMERIC

Turmeric (*Curcuma longa*) is a traditional spice in Indian cuisine; it's what gives curry its color. Its most active constituent, curcumin, has potent anti-inflammatory properties — perhaps the strongest of all the medicinal herbs'. Its efficacy has been compared to NSAIDs and other anti-inflammatory drugs discussed in chapter 6. We do not know exactly how curcumin exerts its anti-inflammatory action, but it is believed that it may work like corticosteroids.

Turmeric is very safe, with no adverse side effects or toxicity. The best turmeric preparations are standardized for curcumin, and the recommended dose is 200 mg once or twice a day.

FEVERFEW

Feverfew (*Tanacetum parthenium*), as you might guess, has been used traditionally for fever. However, the most common use for this member of the chrysanthemum family today is in the treatment of the pain of migraine headache and arthritis. The active ingredients in feverfew, sesquiterpene lactones and parthenolides, obstruct the production of prostaglandins, thereby alleviating pain and inflammation. Feverfew also inhibits the production of an inflammatory component in white blood cells, a special concern in rheumatoid arthritis and other autoimmune diseases. Although feverfew may not knock out a full-blown migraine headache, taking it preventively on a daily basis over a period of several weeks to months is effective in decreasing the incidence of migraines.

Look for a product with standardized extracts of sesquiterpene lactones (100 mcg) and parthenolides (400 mcg), and take one a day.[19]

GINGER

Ginger (*Zingiber officinale*) is a popular, pungent culinary spice, as well as a component of many Chinese herbal preparations. Fresh gingerroot or ginger supplements relieve the morning sickness common in early pregnancy and prevent motion sickness. In addition, ginger is a powerful anti-inflammatory, acting like several of the herbs cited above, as well as NSAIDs, on inflammatory prostaglandin pathways. Try fresh ginger or 100 mg supplements.

LET FOOD BE YOUR MEDICINE

A healthy diet and comprehensive nutritional supplement program are requisites for optimal health, even for the healthiest of us — and their importance is even more pronounced if you're suffering with pain. In most cases your choices of food are not going to cure your pain overnight (although eliminating food allergens has been known to). But proper nutrition *will* put you on the path to better health and increase your resistance and your rebound time. And some of the nutritional supplements and herbal remedies discussed in this chapter are useful adjuncts to magnet therapy for pain relief.

Chapter Eleven

PUTTING IT ALL TOGETHER: THE FUTURE OF MAGNET THERAPY

Using magnets on the surface of the skin for pain relief is an effective, exciting, and, we're happy to say, developing field. As we indicated in chapter 5, each person who works with magnets has his or her own ideas as to how and why magnets work, and they are quite divergent. New treatment possibilities are always subject to speculation as well as disbelief, like the varying theories that surfaced when TENS and acupuncture began to be used to help control pain.

Questions about the hows and whys of the success of static magnetic field therapy for pain relief are now closer than ever to being answered fully. We hope we've answered a few in this book. Likely, we've raised more, and that's okay, too.

Like seeds in the wind, there are plenty of anecdotal stories floating around about the effect of magnets on soft tissue and on musculoskeletal injuries; they tell us that the field is ripe for potential growth. But more well-controlled studies are also needed.

Often the person or company recounting these circulating stories has a financial interest in the magnet industry. Yet many of the doctors involved with these companies got into the field because someone in their family was experiencing pain that no other medical procedure could relieve. And like a spreading American folk remedy, "someone recommended they use magnets." Skeptics at first, they stayed to applaud, to use them on themselves, and even to alter their practice to incorporate magnets.

Well-controlled studies that use proper research procedures are precisely what is needed at this point, but for the time being we must be satisfied with less than total scientific evidence. Even as we write this, double-blind studies are under way.

At this point, the lack of a good database of well-controlled studies puts magnet therapy, for some, in the realm of quackery, as happens in any emerging new field. And we would be the first to admit, there's quackery out there. There's also titillatingly suggestive evidence to indicate that magnet therapy works, and works better than some more expensive therapies.

We've distinguished for you the difference between pulsed electromagnetic fields generated by electric coils and static magnetic fields, the difference between electromagnets and permanent magnets. We've showed you that in many ways the field is not new; the use of magnets, and the belief in their effectiveness, has been with us for a long time.

We've shared with you some of the successful personal experiences of not only famous athletes whose profession subjects them to intense and continuous physical strain, but also ordinary people with the everyday kinds of pains you and I have. Magnets work for both.

We are not advocating that magnet therapy replace the conventional treatment for serious illnesses like cancer, diabetes, and cardiac disease. We do believe that it may relieve the pains associated with those disorders and serve as a valuable accompaniment to conventional medicine. As we indicated in chapter 6, magnets may very well reduce the need for anti-inflammatory drugs, and thereby lower the risks of various drug-related side effects. Nor are we advocating that you use magnets instead of consulting a doctor. You run the risk of not finding a serious illness that could be treated before it's too late.

What magnets cannot do is improve the ultimate state of your health in the manner that nutrition and exercise can. Again, magnets may allow you to feel better before, during, and after exercise, but they can't take the place of it for long-term health benefits. They won't take the place of adequate and proper nutrition; however, they may make you feel well enough that you desire to eat better to live longer (where once, perhaps, the pain was so intense that you didn't care).

Magnets are one important part of a holistic therapy that affects the entire mind–body interaction. With almost 33 million Americans functionally limited in their daily activities by some form of chronic pain, new, multifaceted approaches have to be considered.[1] And we believe that we have amply demonstrated why magnetic field therapy can be an important adjunct to those approaches.

There's room, and a need, for much research here, as there is with any new medical approach. Some of the questions we have include:

1. Which kinds of magnets work best for which kinds of pain?
2. How do magnets work when used in conjunction with mind–body techniques already shown to be effective, such as physiotherapy and biofeedback?
3. What are the long-term and short-term effects of magnets? How often does pain reoccur with magnets? (We've heard anecdotal stories that run the gamut from never having to use the magnets again to having to use them occasionally with a flare-up.)

4. We're sorry to say that magnets appear to be ineffective for some people — so we've been told by them. Why? Does it relate to their belief system, their psychosocial characteristics, or, possibly, to differences in their physiological make-up?

SUMMING IT UP

An old Chinese proverb says that if the birds of worry fly around your head, you can't help that, but if they nest there, you can. In other words, you may not be able to live totally pain free, but you can certainly refuse to let pain take over your life. You can shoo those birds out and find positive ways to cope with pain.

Psychologists say that what we tell ourselves about what we can or cannot do more strongly influences what we actually can do than our actual capabilities. We do know that our perception of the environment (the people, places, and things we encounter), our individual interpretation or understanding of it, determines the kinds of experiences we have. We filter out what we don't expect to see and focus on what our personal bias or attitude predetermines us to see — and having seen it, we are once again justified in holding on to our attitude. Attitudes, however, are learned. They aren't put in place while we're in the womb; they are not genetic and they are not inherited.

In terms of pain management, this means that even if you learned your attitudes toward pain, disability, capability, diet, and exercise long ago, you have the ability — and opportunity — to learn new, more effective ones. We also bet that magnets weren't part of that old learning — how could they be? — so you have two choices there. You can say your family didn't use them, so you aren't going to either. Or you can say, "A new opportunity! I'll check this out and see how it works for me."

The integration of magnets with both conventional and alternative approaches to medicine faces a bright future. There are exciting new therapeutic procedures to be developed and researched. We see this as

THE END . . . AND THE BEGINNING

And as we track the developments of magnet therapy, so can you by logging on to Brenda Adderly's website at www.BrendaAdderly.com, and by reading her monthly newsletter (888-211-2800). Dr. Whitaker's monthly newsletter, *Health & Healing* (800-539-8219), will also keep you up to date on the latest developments in magnets and other safe, effective therapeutic modalities.

NOTES

Introduction

1. Kyoichi Nakagawa. "Magnetic Field Deficiency Syndrome and Magnetic Treatment." Translation of an article that appeared in *Japan Medical Journal,* Dec. 4, 1976, 2745.

2. L. Kuritzky, "Death, Taxes, and Acute Low Back Pain." *Hospital Practice* (office edition), 29(11) (Nov. 15, 1994): 53–54.

3. V. Mooney, "What Is Going to Happen to Back Pain?" *Journal of the Royal Society of Medicine,* 86 (1993): 273–76.

4. From information supplied by the Back Pain Association of America. For additional information, contact them at P.O. Box 135, Pasadena, MD 21123-0136, tel. (410) 255-7392.

Chapter 1: WHAT EXACTLY *IS* MAGNETISM?

1. George Washins and Richard Hricak, *Discovery of Magnetic Health* (Rockville, Md.: Nova Publishing, 1993), p. 200.

2. R. O. Becker, *Cross Currents: The Promise of Electromedicine; The Perils of Electropollution* (New York: Tarcher/Putnam, 1990), 70.

3. H. Hannemann, *Magnet Therapy* (New York: Sterling, 1990), 17.

Chapter 2: THE HISTORY OF MAGNET THERAPY

1. Jwing-Ming Yang, *Chinese Quigong Massage* (Hong Kong: Yang's Martial Arts Association, 1992), 14.

2. Washnis and Hricak, *Discovery of Magnetic Health,* 46.

3. James Livingston, *Driving Force: The Natural Magic of Magnets* (Cambridge, Mass.: Harvard University Press, 1996), 14.

4. Becker, *Cross Currents,* 17.

5. Ibid., 18.

6. Robert O. Becker and Gary Selden, *The Body Electric* (New York: Morrow, 1985), 245–54.

7. K. Thomas, *Religion and the Decline of Magic* (New York: Scribners, 1971), 222.

8. E. Ashmole, *Theatrum Chemicum Brittannicum* (1652; reprint, Kessinyer Publishing, 1997), 464.

9. Livingston, *Driving Force,* 29.

10. W. S. Kroger, *Clinical and Experimental Hypnosis* (Philadelphia: Lippincott, 1963), 1–2.

11. L. R. Wolberg, *Medical Hypnosis,* vol. 1, *The Principles of Hypnotherapy* (New York: Grune & Stratton, 1948), 1–3.

12. Quoted in Livingston, *Driving Force,* 205.

13. Ibid., 204.

14. E. T. Carlson and M. M. Simpson, "Perkinism vs. Mesmerism," *Journal of the History of Behavioral Science* 6 (1970): 16–24.

15. E. R. Hilgard and J. R. Hilgard, *Hypnosis in the Relief of Pain* (Los Altos, Calif.: Kaufmann, 1975), 2–4.

16. Kroger, *Clinical and Experimental Hypnosis,* 2.

17. F. H. Frankel, *Hypnosis: Trance as a Coping Mechanism* (New York: Plenum, 1976), 6.

18. Livingston, *Driving Force,* 206.

19. Frankel, *Hypnosis,* 9.

20. Livingston, *Driving Force,* 209.

21. Heinz Schiegl, *Healing Magnetism* (York Beach, Maine: Samuel Weiser, 1987), 25.

22. J. M. Quen, "Elisha Perkins, Physician, Nostrum-Vendor, or Charlatan?" *Bulletin of the History of Medicine* 27 (1963): 159–66.

23. Ibid., 162.

24. Livingston, *Driving Force,* 208.

25. Ibid., 209.

26. Ibid., 212.

27. Becker, *Cross Currents,* 81.

Chapter 3: MAGNETS WORK

1. W. R. Adey, "Our Changing Electromagnetic Environment: A Century of Rewards and New Responsibilities as We Fashion a Most Precious Asset to Our Needs" (Paper presented at the Ninth International Montreux Congress on Stress, Montreux, Switzerland, Feb. 16–21, 1997).

2. E. R. Sanseverino, A. Vannini, and P. Castellaci, "Therapeutic Effects of Pulsed Magnetic Fields on Joint Diseases," *Panminerva Med* 34, no. 4 (1992): 187–96.

3. D. Foley-Nolan, C. Barry, R. J. Coughlin, P. O'Connor, and D. Roden, "Pulsed High Frequency (27 MHz) Electromagnetic Therapy for Persistent Neck Pain: A Double-Blind, Placebo-Controlled Study of 20 Patients," *Orthopedics* 13, no. 4 (April 1990): 445–51.

4. R. Sandyk, K. Derpapas, P. A. Anninos, and N. Tsagas, "Magnetic Fields in the Treatment of Parkinson's Disease," *International Journal of Neuroscience* 63 (1992): 141–50.

5. R. Sandyk, "Rapid Normalization of Visual Evoked Potentials of Picotesla Range Magnetic Fields in Chronic Progressive Multiple Sclerosis," *International Journal of Neuroscience* 77 (1994): 243–59.

6. Mark George, E. Wasserman, W. Williams, A. Callahan, T. A. Ketter, P. Basser, M. Hallett, and R. M. Post, "Daily Repetitive

Transcranial Magnetic Stimulation (or TMS) Improves Mood in Depression," *NeuroReport* 6, no. 14 (Oct. 2, 1995): 1853–56.

7. V. V. Kuz'menko and Y. D. Katz, "Magnetic Field in the Treatment of Pain Syndromes of the Stumps of the Extremities," *Ortopedia Travmatologia I Protezir Ovanie* 6 (June 1982): 8–12.

8. D. M. Long, S. Uematsu, and R. B. Kouba, "Placebo Responses to Medical Device Therapy for Pain," *Stereotact Functional Neurosurgery* 53, no. 3 (1989): 149–56.

9. A. Binder, G. Parr, B. Hazelman, and S. Fitton-Jackson, "Pulsed Electromagnetic Field Therapy of Persistent Rotator Cuff Tendinitis," *Lancet,* March 31, 1984, 695–98.

10. B. Rubink, R. O. Becker, R. G. Flower, C. F. Hazelwood, A. R. Liboff, and J. Walleczek, "Alternative Medicine: Expanding Medical Horizons." Presentation paper, 1992.

11. I. Mulay and L. N. Mulay, "Effect of Magnetic Field on Sarcoma 37 Ascites Tumour Cells," *Nature,* June 10, 1961, 1019.

12. M. F. Barnothy, "Biological Effects of Magnetic Fields on Small Mammals," *BioMedical Sciences Instrumentation* 1 (1963): 127–35.

13. D. B. Tata, N. F. Vanhouten, E. Brook, and T. R. Triton, "Non-Invasive, Permanent Magnetic Field Modality Induces Lethal Effects on Several Rodent and Human Cancers," *Proceedings of the American Association for Cancer Research* 35 (March 1994): 386.

14. R. L. Raylman, A. C. Clavo, and R. L. Wahl, "Exposure to Strong Static Magnetic Field Slows the Growth of Human Cancer Cells in Vitro," *Bioelectromagnetics* 17 (1996): 358–63.

15. R. Rogachefsky, "Use of Tectonic Magnet for Treatment of Hand after Gun Shot," *North American Academy of Magnetic Therapy Newsletter* 1, no. 1 (1997).

16. C. Takeshige and M. Sato, "Comparison of Pain Relief Mechanisms Between Needling to the Muscle, Static Magnetic Field,

External *Qigong* and Needling to the Acupuncture Point," *Acupuncture and Electro-Therapeutics Research* 21, no. 2 (April 1996): 119–31.

17. J. P. Prince, "The Use of Low Strength Magnets on EAV Points," *American Journal of Acupuncture* 3, no. 2 (1983): 125–30.

18. D. W. Harper and E. F. Wright, "Magnets as Analgesics," *Lancet,* July 2, 1977, 47.

19. J. B. Baron, Y. Rocard, H. Fukushima, J. C. Bessineton, G. Bizzo, and S. Takahashi, "Interaction Between Labyrinthine Electrical Mechanical Stimulations and Musculo-Oculo-Nucal Magnetic Stimulation on Tonic Postural Activity" (Paper presented at the Seventh International Symposium of the International Society of Posturography, Houston, Texas, 1983).

20. K. S. Kim and Y. J. Lee, "The Effect of Magnetic Application for Primary Dysmenorrhea," *Kanhohak Tamgu* 3, no. 1 (1994): 148–73.

21. E. A. Stepanov, A. P. Erokhin, V. V. Nikolaev, G. S. Vasil'ev, and S. B. Mukho, "Treatment of Short Urethral Strictures in Children Using Magnets," *Ural Nefral* (Mosk) 3 (1989): 8–11.

22. E. Z. Rabinovich, IuP Taran, M. D. Usacheva, and I. M. Epshtein, "Effect of a Constant Magnetic Field on the Respiration of Human Skin During Reparative and Destructive Processes," *An. Kuznetsov. Biolizika* 28, no. 4 (1983): 693–96.

23. A. Weinberger, A. Nyska, and S. Giler, "Treatment of Experimental Inflammatory Synovitis with Continuous Magnetic Field," *Israel Journal of Medical Science* 32, no. 12 (1966): 1197–1201.

Chapter 4: PERMANENT MAGNETS ARE SAFE

1. J. E. Eiselein, H. M. Bontell, and M. W. Biggs, "Biological Effects of Magnetic Fields — Negative Results," *Aerospace Medicine,* May 1961, 383–86.

2. E. Hall, J. Bedford, and M. J. M. Leask, "Some Negative Results in the Search for a Lethal Effect of Magnetic Fields on Biological Materials," *Nature* 203 (Sept. 5, 1964), 1086–87.

3. G. Ardito, L. Lamberti, P. Bigatti, and G. Prono, "Influence of a Constant Magnetic Field on Human Lymphocyte Cultures," *Societa Italione Di Bolognia Sperimentale* 60(7-12), 1984.

4. A. E. Greene and M. H. Halpern, "Response of Tissue Culture Cells to Low Magnetic Fields," *Aerospace Medicine* 37, no. 3 (March 1966): 251–53.

5. *Environmental Health Criteria 69 Magnetic Fields* (Geneva: World Health Organization, 1987), 28.

Chapter 5: HOW MAGNET THERAPY WORKS

1. William H. Philpott, W. H. Taplin, and S. Taplin, *Biomagnetic Handbook* (Choctaw, Okla.: Enviro-Tech Products, 1990), 24–25.

2. V. Warnke, "Ultra-Red Radiation and the Partial Pressure of Connective Tissue in Man Seen as an Index of the Effects of Intermittent Magnetic Fields," *Proceedings of the Second International Congress on Magneto-medicine* (Rome, November 8–9, 1980), 17–22.

3. W. C. Cheong, and C. P. Yang, *Synopsis of Chinese Acupuncture,* rev. ed. (Hong Kong: Light Publishing, 1978).

4. D. L. Kirsch, *The Complete Clinical Guide to Electro-Acutherapy,* 2d ed. (Glendale, Calif.: National Electro-Acutherapy Foundation, 1978).

5. T. M. Murphy and J. J. Bonica, "Acupuncture Analgesia and Anesthesia," *Archives of Surgery* 112 (1977): 896–902.

6. Kirsch, *Complete Clinical Guide,* 5.

7. S. Palos, *The Chinese Art of Healing* (New York: Bantam, 1972).

8. S. T. Chang, *The Complete Book of Acupuncture* (Berkeley, Calif.: Celestial Arts, 1976), 21.

9. Cheong and Yang, *Synopsis of Chinese Acupuncture.*

10. Chang, *Complete Book of Acupuncture,* 23.

11. R. P. Steiner, "Acupuncture Cultural Perspectives," *Postgraduate Medicine* 14, no. 4 (1983): 61–62.

12. M. Hallett and L. G. Cohen, "Magnetism: A New Method for Stimulation of Nerve and Brain," *JAMA* 262, no. 4 (July 28, 1989): 538–41.

13. M. J. McLean, R. R. Holcomb, A. W. Wanill, J. D. Pickett, and A. V. Cavopol, "Blockade of Sensory Neuron Action Potentials by a Static Magnetic Field in the 10 mT Range," *Bioelectromagnetics* 16 (1993): 20–32.

14. R. Sandyk, "The Influence of Pineal Gland on Migraine and Cluster Headaches and Effects of Treatment with Picotesla Magnetic Fields," *International Journal of Neuroscience* 67 (1992): 145–71.

15. A. Lerchl, K. O. Honaka, and R. J. Reiter, "Pineal Gland 'Magnetosensitivity' to Static Magnetic Fields Is a Consequence of Induced Electric Currents (Eddy Currents)," *Journal of Pineal Research* 10 (1991): 109–16.

16. G. Kroeker, D. Parkinson, J. Vriend, and J. Peeling, "Neurochemical Effects of Static Magnetic Field Exposure," *Surgical Neuralgia* 45 (1996): 62–66.

17. I. Rosenfeld, *Dr. Rosenfeld's Guide to Alternative Medicine: What Works, What Doesn't — And What's Right for You* (New York: Random House, 1996), 257–60.

18. Takeshige and Sato, "Comparisons of Pain Relief Mechanisms."

Chapter 6: MEDICATIONS

1. B. Stimmel, *Pain, Analgesia, and Addiction: The Pharmacologic Treatment of Pain* (New York: Raven Press, 1983), 1.

2. D. Bowsher, "Acute and Chronic Pain and Assessment," in *Pain Management by Physical Therapy*, 2d ed., ed. P. E. Wells, V. Frampton, and D. Bowsher (Oxford, England: Butterworth-Heinemann, 1994), 39.

3. G. Park and B. Fulton, *The Management of Acute Pain* (Oxford: Oxford University Press, 1991).

4. D. Wright, S. Barrow, A. D. Fisher, S. D. Horsley, and M. I. Jason, "Influence of Physical, Psychological and Behavioural Factors on Consultations for Back Pain," *British Journal of Rheumatology* 34, no. 2 (1995): 156–61.

5. A. M. Unruh, "Gender Variations in Clinical Pain Experience," *Pain* 65, 1996, nos. 2–3, 123–67.

6. E. C. Huskisson, "Pain: Mechanisms and Measurement," in *The Treatment of Chronic Pain*, ed. F. Dudley Hart (Lancaster, England: MTP Medical and Technical Publishing, 1974), 1–38.

7. P. M. Cinciripini, "The Influence of External Information on Judgments of Pain," *Behavior Modification* 19, no. 3 (July 1995): 290–306.

8. J. T. Simms, "Management Strategies for the Chronic Headache Patient," *Pain Management* 4, no. 5 (1991): 17–24.

9. A. Mauskop, "Headaches," in *A Practical Approach to Pain Management*, ed. M. Lefkowitz and A. H. Lebovits, with D. J. Wlody and S. A. Rubin (Boston: Little, Brown, 1996), 233–38.

10. A. Srikiatkhachorn and K. Phanthumchinda, "Prevalence and Clinical Features of Chronic Daily Headache in a Headache Clinic," *Headache* 37 (1997): 277–80.

11. Statistics from foreign countries translated and reported in L.-A. Pini, M. Bigarelli, G. Vitale, and E. Sternieri, "Headaches Associated with Chronic Use of Analgesics: A Therapeutic Approach," *Headache* 36 (1996): 433–39.

12. R. M. Gallagher, "Proper Use of Analgesics in the Treatment of Headache," *Headache Quarterly* 3(1 Suppl) (1992): 22–27.

13. Pini et al., "Headaches Associated with Chronic Use of Analgesics."

14. "The Use of Narcotics in the Treatment of Headache," editorial, *Headache Quarterly* 4, no. 2 (1993): 143–44.

15. N. Lester, J. C. Lefebvre, and F. J. Keefe, "Pain in Young Adults: I. Relationship to Gender and Family Pain History," *Clinical Journal of Pain* 10, no. 4 (1994): 282–89.

16. K. L. Casey, "Introduction to Section B: An Overview of the Neurological Significance of Pain," in *Mechanisms of Pain and Analgesic Compounds,* ed. R. F. Beers, Jr., and E. G. Bassett (New York: Raven Press, 1979), 107.

17. C. R. Chapman, "Contribution of Research on Acupunctural and Transcutaneous Electrical Stimulation to the Understanding of Pain Mechanisms and Pain Relief," in *Mechanisms of Pain and Analgesic Compounds,* 71.

18. N. Lester, et al., "Pain in Young Adults."

19. C. Hultman, M. Nordin, and H. Saraste, "Physical and Psychological Workload in Men with and Without Low Back Pain," *Scandinavian Journal of Rehabilitative Medicine* 27, no. 1 (1995): 11–17.

20. I. Foppa and R. H. Noack, "The Relation of Self-Reported Back Pain to Psychosocial, Behavioral, and Health-Related Factors in a Working Population in Switzerland," *Social Science and Medicine* 43, no. 7 (1996): 1119–26.

21. J. Slack, and M. Faut-Callahan, "Pain Management," *Nursing Clinics of North America* 26, no. 2 (1991): 463–76.

22. K. Ghose, "Pain and the Elderly," in *Drug Management of Pain in the Elderly*, ed. K. Ghose (Lancaster, England: MTP Press, 1987), 1–7.

23. R. T. Goldberg, "Childhood Abuse, Depression, and Chronic Pain," *Clinical Journal of Pain* 19, no. 4: 277–81.

24. J. Gomez, "Psychological Aspects of Pain," in *Drug Management of Pain in the Elderly*, 9–16.

25. I. Pilowsky, "Abnormal Illness Behavior," *British Journal of Medical Psychology* 42 (1969): 347–51.

26. S. J. Eisendrath, "Psychiatric Aspects of Chronic Pain," *Neurology* 45 (12 Suppl 9) (1995): S26–S34.

27. R. McIndoe, "A Behavioral Approach to the Management of Chronic Pain: A Self Management Perspective," *The Australian Family Physician* 23, 1994, no. 12, 2284–92.

28. B. Aghabeigi, "The Pathophysiology of Pain," *British Dental Journal* 173, no. 8 (1992): 91–97.

29. B. J. Lister, "Dilemmas in the Treatment of Chronic Pain," *American Journal of Medicine*, 101(Suppl. 1A) (July 31, 1996): 2S–5S.

30. J. A. Markenson, "Mechanism of Chronic Pain," *American Journal of Medicine* 101 (Suppl. 1A) (July 31, 1996), 6S–18S.

31. G. E. Ruoff, "Chronic Pain in Primary Care," *Headache Quarterly* 6, no. 1 (1995): 19–25.

32. S. A. King, "Psychological Aspects of Pain," *Mount Sinai Journal of Medicine* 58, no. 3 (1991): 203–207.

33. J. J. Bonica, "Important Clinical Aspects of Acute and Chronic Pain," in *Mechanisms of Pain and Analgesic Compounds*, 15–29.

34. Ruoff, "Chronic Pain in Primary Care."

35. A. H. Lebovits and L. E. Bassman, "Psychological Aspects of

Chronic Pain," in *A Practical Approach to Pain Management,* 124–28.

36. J. Schofferman, "Long-Term Use of Opioid Analgesics for the Treatment of Chronic Pain of Nonmalignant Origin," *Journal of Pain Symptom Management* 8, no. 5 (1993): 279–88.

37. Ibid.

38. Long et al., "Placebo Responses."

39. M. A. Lumley, T. Torosian, M. W. Ketterer, and S. D. Pickard, "Psychosocial Factors Related to Noncardiac Chest Pain During Treadmill Exercise," *Psychosomatics* 38, no. 3 (1997): 230–38.

40. R. McIndoe, *Op. cit.*

41. J. Schofferman, "Long-Term Use of Opioid Analgesics."

42. R. Melzack and P. D. Wall, "Pain Mechanisms: A New Theory," *Science* 150 (1965): 971–79.

43. R. Melzack and S. G. Dennis, "Pain Mechanisms: Theoretical Approaches," in *Mechanisms of Pain and Analgesic Compounds,* 185–93.

44. R. E. Wilson, "Transcutaneous Electrical Nerve Stimulation," in *A Practical Approach to Pain Management,* 136–41.

45. Park and Fulton, *Management of Acute Pain,* 19.

46. "Editorial: Update on Opioid Receptors," *British Journal of Anaesthesiology* 73, no. 2 (1994): 132–34.

47. L. E. Mather and M. J. Cousins, "The Pharmacological Relief of Pain — Contemporary Issues," *Medical Journal of Australia* 156, no. 11 (1992): 796–802.

48. J. T. Cannon and J. C. Liebeskind, "Descending Control Systems," in *Mechanisms of Pain and Analgesic Compounds,* 171–84.

49. R. E. Wilson, "Transcutaneous Electrical Nerve Stimulation," in *A Practical Approach to Pain Management,* 136–41.

50. D. Griffiths, *Psychology and Medicine* (London: Macmillan, 1980).

51. A. A. Petrie, *Individuality in Pain and Suffering* (Chicago: University of Chicago Press, 1967).

52. S. G. B. Eysenck, 1961 study cited in S. French, "The Psychology and Sociology of Pain," in *Pain Management by Physical Therapy,* 2d ed., ed. P. E. Wells, V. Frampton, and D. Bowsher (Oxford: Butterworth-Heinemann, 1994), 17–28.

53. N. Lester et al., "Pain in Young Adults."

54. M. Knaster, *Discovering the Body's Wisdom* (New York: Bantam, 1996), 99.

55. R. M. Pearson, "Non-steroidal Anti-Inflammatory Drugs," in *Drug Management of Pain in the Elderly,* 39–44.

56. D. M. Richlin, "Nonnarcotic Analgesics and Tricyclic Antidepressants for the Treatment of Chronic Nonmalignant Pain," *Mount Sinai Journal of Medicine* 58, no. 3 (1991): 221–28.

57. N. M. Agrawal, "What Explains NSAID Gastropathy?" *Journal of Musculoskeletal Medicine* 8, no. 9 (1991): 31–37.

58. S. H. Roth, "Nonsteroidal Anti-Inflammatory Drugs: Gastropathy, Deaths, and Medical Practice," *Annals of Internal Medicine* 109 (1988): 353–54.

59. D. J. Bjorkman, "Nonsteroidal Anti-Inflammatory Drug–Induced Gastrointestinal Injury," *American Journal of Medicine* 101 Suppl. 1A (July 31, 1996): 25S–31S.

60. M. Sosnowski, "Pathophysiology of Acute Pain," *Pain Digest* 4, no. 2 (1994): 100–105.

61. P. W. Baumert, Jr., "Acute Inflammation After Injury: Quick Control Speeds Rehabilitation," *Postgraduate Medicine* 97, no. 2 (1995): 35–36.

62. Park and Fulton, *Management of Acute Pain.*

63. C. P. N. Watson, "Antidepressant Drugs as Adjuvant Anal-
    gesics," *Journal of Pain Symptom Management* 9, no. 6 (1994):
    392–405.

64. Ibid.

65. N. C. Maruyama and W. Breitbart, "Psychotropic Adjuvant
    Analgesics for Chronic Pain," in *A Practical Approach to Pain
    Management*, 41–61.

66. Stimmel, *Pain, Analgesia, and Addiction*, 207.

67. Ibid., 250.

68. S. Begley, "Jagged Little Pill," *Newsweek*, August 18, 1997, 66.

69. Stimmel, *Pain, Analgesia, and Addiction*, 69.

70. S. Begley, "Jagged Little Pill."

71. J. Feltman, ed., *Prevention's Food & Nutrition* (Emmaus, Pa.: Ro-
    dale Press, 1993), 64.

72. K. Butler and L. Rayner, *The New Handbook of Health and Pre-
    ventive Medicine* (Buffalo, N.Y.: Prometheus Books, 1990), 333.

73. H. Merksey, "Pharmacological Approaches Other Than Opioids
    in Chronic Non-Cancer Pain Management," *Acta Anaesthesio-
    logica Scandinavica* 41, no. 1 (pt. 2) (1997): 187–90.

74. G. Bronfort, C. H. Goldsmith, C. F. Nelson, P. D. Boline, and A. V.
    Anderson, "Trunk Exercise Combined with Spinal Manipulative
    or NSAID Therapy for Chronic Low Back Pain: A Randomized,
    Observer-Blinded Clinical Trial," *Journal of Manipulative and
    Physiological Therapeutics* 19, no. 9 (1996): 570–82.

75. Stimmel, *Pain, Analgesia, and Addiction*, 83.

76. V. B. Saladini, Jr., "Nonsteroidal Anti-inflammatory Drugs," in
    A Practical Approach to Pain Management, 27–31.

77. Butler and Rayner, *New Handbook*, 333.

78. Ghose, "Drug Management of Pain in the Elderly," 1–7.

79. H. L. Rosner, "The Pharmacologic Management of Acute Post-operative Pain," in *A Practical Approach to Pain Management,* 5–14.

80. Butler and Rayner, *New Handbook,* 131.

81. N. M. Agrawal, "What Explains NSAID Gastropathy?" *Journal of Musculoskeletal Medicine* 8, no. 9 (1991): 31–37.

82. C. L. Bartels, "Nonsteroidal Anti-Inflammatory Drugs in Acute Pain Management," *Journal of Pharmaceutical Care and Pain Symptom Control* 1, no. 3 (1993): 21–38.

83. M. C. Allison, A. G. Howatson, C. J. Torrance, F. D. Lee, and R. I. Russell, "Gastrointestinal Damage Associated with the Use of Nonsteroidal Antiinflammatory Drugs," *New England Journal of Medicine* 327, no. 11 (1992): 749–54.

84. J. H. Yost and G. R. Morgan, Jr., "Cardiovascular Effects of NSAIDs," *Journal of Musculoskeletal Medicine* 11, no. 10 (1994): 22–34.

85. Saladini, "Nonsteroidal Anti-Inflammatory Drugs"; R. M. Pearson, "Non-Steroidal Anti-Inflammatory Drugs," in *Drug Management of Pain in the Elderly,* 43.

86. Ibid., 39–44.

87. S. F. Brena and S. H. Sanders, "Opioids in Nonmalignant Pain: Questions in Search of Answers," *Clinical Journal of Pain* 7, no. 4 (1991): 342–45.

88. Park and Fulton, *Management of Acute Pain,* 34.

89. R. L. Brown, M. F. Fleming, and J. J. Patterson, "Chronic Opioid Analgesic Therapy for Chronic Low Back Pain," *Journal of the American Board of Family Practice* 9, no. 3 (1996): 191–204.

90. Stimmel, *Pain, Analgesia, and Addiction,* 106.

91. J. A. Henry, "Clinical Pharmacology of the Narcotic Analgesics," in *Drug Management of Pain in the Elderly,* 27–38.

NOTES

Chapter 7: HOW TO USE MAGNETS TO TREAT YOUR SPECIFIC PAIN

1. Coauthor Brenda Adderly has set up a website where a summary of this study, as well as other up-to-date information on magnet therapy and other matters pertaining to personal and family wellness, can be found. The website address is www.BrendaAdderly.com.
2. Daniel Man, Boris Man, Harvey Plosker, and Marko Markov, "Effect of Permanent Magnetic Field on Postoperative Pain and Wound Healing in Plastic Surgery" (Paper presented at the Second World Congress on Electricity and Magnetism in Biology and Medicine, Bologna, Italy, June 8–13, 1997).
3. Becker and Selden, *The Body Electric: Electromagnetism and the Foundation of Life.*
4. E. J. Rogers and R. J. Rogers, "Tension-Type Headaches, Fibromyalgia, or Myofascial Pain," *Headache Quarterly* 2, no. 4 (1991): 273–77.
5. B. E. Benjamin, *Listen to Your Pain: The Active Person's Guide to Understanding, Identifying, and Treating Pain and Injury* (New York: Penguin, 1984), 7.
6. G. W. Jay, "Sympathetic Aspects of Myofascial Pain," *Pain Digest* 5, no. 4 (1995): 192–94.
7. Melzack and Dennis, "Pain Mechanisms," 189.

Chapter 8: EXERCISE THAT HELPS, NOT HURTS

1. M. Campello, M. Nordin, and S. Weiser, "Physical Exercise and Low Back Pain," *Scandinavian Journal of Medicine and Science in Sports* 6, no. 2 (1996): 63–72.

199

2. McIndoe, R., "A Behavioral Approach to the Management of Chronic Pain: A Self Management Perspective," *The Australian Family Physician* 23, no. 12 (1994), 2284–92.

3. B. W. Nelson, E. O'Reilly, M. Miller, M. Hogan, J. A. Wegner, and C. Kelly, "The Clinical Effects of Intensive, Specific Exercise on Chronic Low Back Pain: A Controlled Study of 895 Consecutive Patients with 1-Year Follow-Up," *Orthopedics* 18, no. 10 (1995): 971–81.

4. A. Pace, "How to Develop the Exercise Habit," *Bottom Line Health* 11, no. 8 (August 1997): 13–14.

5. McIndoe, R. *Op. cit.*

6. A. C. King, R. F. Oman, G. S. Brassington, D. L. Bliwise, and W. L. Haskell, "Moderate-Intensity Exercise and Self-Rated Quality of Sleep in Older Adults: A Randomized Controlled Trial," *JAMA* 277, no. 1 (Jan. 1, 1997): 32–37. See also N. A. Singh, K. M. Clements, and M. A. Fiatarone, "A Randomized Controlled Trial of the Effect of Exercise on Sleep," *Sleep* 29, no. 2 (1997): 95–101.

7. A. W. Sedgwick, M. J. Davies, and D. S. Smith, "Changes Over Four Years in Musculoskeletal Impairment in Men and Women," *Medical Journal of Australia* 161, no. 8 (1994): 482–86.

8. G. E. Schwartz, R. J. Davidson, and D. J. Goleman, "Patterning of Cognitive and Somatic Processes in the Self-Regulation of Anxiety: Effects of Meditation Versus Exercise," *Psychosomatic Medicine* 40, no. 4 (1978): 321–28.

9. I. Vuori, "Exercise and Physical Health: Musculoskeletal Health and Functional Capabilities," *Research Quarterly for Exercise and Sport* 66, no. 4 (1995): 276–85.

10. D. T. Lowenthal, D. A. Kirschener, N. T. Scarpace, M. Pollock,

and J. Graves, "Effects of Exercise on Age and Disease," *Southern Medical Journal* 87, no. 5 (1994): S5–S12.

11. A. Malmivaara, U. Häkkinen, T. Aro, M.-L. Heinrichs, L. Koskenniemi, E. Kuosma, S. Lappi, R. Paloheimo, C. Servo, V. Vaaranen, and S. Hernberg, "The Treatment of Acute Low Back Pain — Bed Rest, Exercises, or Ordinary Activity?" *New England Journal of Medicine* 332, no. 6 (1995): 351–55.

12. E. M. Jenkins and D. G. Borenstein, "Exercise for the Low Back Pain Patient," *Baillieres Clinical Rheumatology* 8, no. 1 (1994): 191–97.

13. R. G. Donelson, "Identifying Appropriate Exercises for Your Low Back Pain Patient," *Journal of Musculoskeletal Medicine* 8, no. 12 (1991): 14–29.

14. T. Kuukkanen and E. Malkia, "Muscular Performance After a 3-Month Progressive Physical Exercise Program and 9-Month Follow-Up in Subjects with Low Back Pain: A Controlled Study," *Scandinavian Journal of Medicine and Science in Sports* 6, no. 2 (1996): 112–21.

15. E. Malkia and A. E. Ljunggren, "Exercise Programs for Subjects with Low Back Disorders," *Scandinavian Journal of Medicine and Science in Sports* 6, no. 2 (1996): 73–81.

16. J. M. Hammill, T. M. Cook, and J. C. Rosecrance, "Effectiveness of a Physical Therapy Regimen in the Treatment of Tension-Type Headache," *Headache* 36, no. 3 (1996): 149–53.

17. W. E. Fordyce, "Principles of Operant Conditioning in Pain Research and Therapy," in *Mechanisms of Pain and Analgesic Compounds,* 85–95.

18. G. Crombez, L. Vervaet, F. Baeyens, R. Lysens, and P. Eelen, "Do Pain Expectancies Cause Pain in Chronic Low Back Patients?

A Clinical Investigation," *Behavior Research and Therapy* 34, no. 11–12 (1996): 919–25.

19. K. Mashima, J. C. Bessineton, and J. B. Baron, "Influence of Permanent Magnetic Field on Tonic Postural Activity," *Medica Physica,* 9 (1986): 37–40.

20. J. B. Bartholomew, B. P. Lewis, D. E. Linder, and D. B. Cook, "Post-Exercise Analgesia: Replication and Extension," *Journal of Sports Sciences* 14, no. 4 (1996): 329–34.

21. K. F. Kolytn, A. W. Garvin, R. L. Gardiner, and T. F. Nelson, "Perception of Pain Following Aerobic Exercise," *Medicine and Science in Sports and Exercise* 28, no. 11 (1996): 1418–21.

22. M. Gurevich, P. M. Kohn, and C. Davis, "Exercise-Induced Analgesia and the Role of Reactivity in Pain Sensitivity," *Journal of Sports Science* 12, no. 6 (Dec. 1994): 549–59.

23. P. A. Dexter, "Joint Exercises in Elderly Persons with Symptomatic Osteoarthritis of the Hip or Knee," *Arthritis Care and Research* 5 (1992): 36–41.

24. G. M. Jensen and C. D. Lorish, "Promoting Patient Cooperation with Exercise Programs: Linking Research, Theory and Practice," *Arthritis Care and Research* (1994) 7, no. 4, 181–87.

25. Butler and Rayner, *New Handbook of Health and Preventive Medicine,* 83.

26. R. B. Arnot, *The Complete Manual of Fitness and Well-Being* (New York: Viking, 1984), 90.

27. V. Simmons and P. D. Hansen, "Effectiveness of Water Exercise on Postural Mobility in the Well Elderly: An Experimental Study on Balance Enhancement," *Journal of Gerontology. Series A, Biological Sciences and Medical Sciences* 51, no. 5 (1996): M233–38.

28. M. S. Templeton, D. L. Booth, and W. D. O'Kelly, "Effects of

Aquatic Therapy on Joint Flexibility and Functional Ability in Subjects with Rheumatic Disease," *Journal of Orthopedic and Sports Physical Therapy* 23, no. 6 (1996): 376–81.

29. *Dorland's Illustrated Medical Dictionary,* 24th ed. (Philadelphia: Saunders, 1965).

30. A. W. Gardner, J. S. Skinner, C. X. Bryant, and L. K. Smith, "Stair Climbing Elicits a Lower Cardiovascular Demand Than Walking in Claudication Patients," *Journal of Cardiopulmonary Rehabilitation* 15, no. 2 (1995): 134–42.

31. For a catalog of workout music audiotapes for different music tastes and fitness levels, contact Sports Music Inc., Box 769689, Roswell, Georgia 30076.

32. Pace, "How to Develop the Exercise Habit," 14.

33. L. E. Grivetti and E. A. Applegate, "From Olympia to Atlanta: A Cultural-Historical Perspective on Diet and Athletic Training," *Journal of Nutrition* 127, no. 5 (1997): 860S–68S.

34. A. J. Guymer, "The Neuromuscular Facilitation of Movement," in *Pain Management by Physical Therapy,* 2d ed., ed. P. E. Wells, V. Frampton, and D. Bowsher (Oxford: Butterworth-Heinemann, 1994), 89–99.

35. W. J. Evans, "Exercise, Nutrition, and Aging," *Journal of Nutrition* 122, no. 3, Suppl. (1992): 796–801.

36. J. M. Schilke, G. O. Johnson, T. J. Housh, and J. R. O'Dell, "Effects of Muscle-Strength Training on the Functional Status of Patients with Osteoarthritis of the Knee Joint," *Nursing Research* 45, no. 2 (1996): 68–72.

37. K. D. Brandt, "Nonsurgical Management of Osteoarthritis, with an Emphasis on Nonpharmacologic Measures," *Archives of Family Medicine* 4, no. 12 (1995): 1057–64.

38. J. F. Reynolds, T. D. Noakes, M. P. Schwellnus, A. Windt, and

P. Bowerbank, "Non-Steroidal Anti-inflammatory Drugs Fail to Enhance Healing of Acute Hamstring Injuries Treated with Physiotherapy," *South African Medical Journal* 85, no. 6 (1995): 517–22.

39. H. Bentsen, F. Lindgarde, and R. Manthorpe, "The Effect of Dynamic Strength Back Exercise and/or a Home Training Program in 57-Year-Old Women with Chronic Low Back Pain: Results of a Prospective Randomized Study with a 3-Year Follow-Up Period," *Spine* 22, no. 13 (1997): 1494–1500.

40. N. A. Singh, K. M. Clements, and M. A. Fiatarone, "A Randomized Controlled Trial of Progressive Resistance Training in Depressed Elders," *Journals of Gerontology: Series A, Biological Sciences and Medical Sciences* 52, no. 1 (1997): M27–35.

41. R. M. Lampman, "Exercise Prescription for Chronically Ill Patients," *American Family Physician* 55, no. 6 (1997): 2185–92.

42. K. Cooper, "Dr. Ken Cooper's Exercise Program for Year-Round Health," *Bottom Line Personal* 18, no. 17 (Sept. 1, 1997): 12–13.

43. Butler and Rayner, *New Handbook,* 95.

44. Ibid., 83.

45. R. Crayhon, *Nutrition Made Simple* (New York: M. Evans and Co., 1994), 133.

46. R. A. Sternbach, *Mastering Pain* (London: Arlington Books, 1987).

Chapter 9: NUTRITIONAL HEALING

1. A. Winter and R. Winter, *Eat Right, Be Right* (New York: St. Martin's, 1988), 6.

2. Butler and Rayner, *New Handbook of Health and Preventive Medicine.*

3. Grivetti and Applegate, "From Olympia to Atlanta."

4. J. M. Kremer, J. Bigauoette, A. V. Michalek, M. A. Timchalk,

L. Lininger, R. I. Rynes, C. Huyck, J. Zieminski, and L. E. Bartholomew, "Effects of Manipulation of Dietary Fatty Acids on Clinical Manifestations of Rheumatoid Arthritis," *Lancet,* Jan. 26, 1985, 184–87.

5. J. Mehta, "Intake of Antioxidants Among American Cardiologists," *American Journal of Cardiology* 79 (June 1, 1997): 1558–60.

6. D. S. Khalsa, "Dr. Dharma Singh Khalsa's Very Simple Secrets of Lifelong Brain Power," *Bottom Line Personal* 18, no. 16 (Aug. 15, 1997): 12.

7. M. A. Bowman and T. L. Schwenk, "Family Medicine," *JAMA* 275, no. 23 (June 19, 1996): 1809–10.

8. Khalsa, "Very Simple Secrets," 11–12.

9. M. de Lorgeril, S. Renaud, N. Marnelle, P. Salen, J. L. Martin, I. Monjaud, J. Guidollet, P. Touboul, and J. Delaye, "Mediterranean Alpha-Linolenic Acid–Rich Diet in Secondary Prevention of Coronary Heart Disease," *Lancet,* June 11, 1994, 1454–59.

10. Crayhon, *Nutrition Made Simple,* 45–47.

11. A. S. Wells and N. W. Read, "Influences of Fat, Energy, and Time of Day on Mood and Performance," *Physiology and Behavior* 59, no. 6 (1996): 1069–76.

12. H. M. Lloyd, P. J. Rogers, D. I. Hedderley, and A. F. Walker, "Acute Effects on Mood and Cognitive Performance of Breakfasts Differing in Fat and Carbohydrate Content," *Appetite* 27, no. 2 (Oct. 1996): 151–64.

13. A. S. Wells, N. W. Read, K. Uvnas-Moberg, and P. Alster, "Influences of Fat and Carbohydrate on Postprandial Sleepiness, Mood, and Hormones," *Physiology and Behavior* 61, no. 5 (May 1997): 679–86.

14. Butler and Rayner, *New Handbook,* 28.

15. Winter and Winter, *Eat Right, Be Right,* 6.

16. Butler and Rayner, 399.

17. J. J. Anderson, P. Rondano, and A. Holmes, "Roles of Diet and Physical Activity in the Prevention of Osteoporosis," *Scandinavian Journal of Rheumatology Supplement* 103 (1996): 65–74.

18. Butler and Rayner, 360.

19. S. Marchand, L. Jinxue, and J. Charest, "Effects of Caffeine on Analgesia from Transcutaneous Electrical Nerve Stimulation," *New England Journal of Medicine* 335, no. 5 (1995): 325–26.

20. "On the Safety of Caffeine as an Analgesic Adjuvant" (editorial), *Headache Quarterly* 5, no. 2 (1994): 125–27.

21. Stimmel, *Pain, Analgesia, and Addiction,* 166.

22. R. S. Kunkel, "Chemical Abuse in the Headache Patient," *Pain Management* 4, no. 4 (1991): 27–31.

23. E. L. H. Spierings, "Headache Caused by Medications and Chemicals," *Headache Quarterly* 3, no. 4 (1992): 403–407.

24. D. R. Brown, J. B. Croft, R. F. Anda, D. H. Barrett, and L. B. Escobedo, "Evaluation of Smoking on the Physical Activity and Depressive Symptoms Relationship," *Medicine and Science in Sports and Exercise* 28, no. 2 (1996): 233–40.

25. W. B. Eriksen, S. Brage, and D. Bruusgaard, "Does Smoking Aggravate Musculoskeletal Pain?" *Scandinavian Journal of Rheumatology* 26, no. 1 (1997): 49–54.

26. D. Wright, S. Barrow, A. D. Fisher, S. D. Horsley, and M. I. Jason, "Influence of Physical, Psychological and Behavioural Factors on Consultations for Back Pain," *British Journal of Rheumatology* 34, no. 2 (1995): 156–61.

27. P. Manninen, H. Riihimak, and M. Heliovaara, "Incidence and

Risk Factors of Low-Back Pain in Middle-Aged Farmers," (*Oxford*) 45, no. 3 (1995): 141–46.

28. Crayhon, *Nutrition Made Simple,* 55.

29. J. Kjeldsen-Kragh et al., "Controlled Trial of Fasting and One-Year Vegetarian Diet in Rheumatoid Arthritis," *Lancet,* Oct. 12, 1991, 899–902.

30. Spierings, "Headache Caused by Medications and Chemicals."

31. Ibid.

Chapter 10: TO SUPPLEMENT OR NOT TO SUPPLEMENT

1. A. L. Bernstein and J. S. Dinesen, "Effects of Pharmacologic Doses of B6 on Carpal Tunnel Syndrome, Electroencephalographic Results and Pain," *Journal of the American College of Nutrition* 12, no. 1 (1993): 73–76.

2. Crayhon, *Nutrition Made Simple,* 106–107.

3. Khalsa, "Very Simple Secrets," 11–12.

4. Crayhon, 112.

5. Winter and Winter, *Eat Right, Be Right,* 57.

6. *Alternative Medicine: Expanding Medical Horizons: A Report to the National Institutes of Health on Alternative Medical Systems and Practices in the United States* (Washington, D.C.: U.S. Government Printing Office, 1992).

7. Winter and Winter, 51.

8. J. Carper, *The Food Pharmacy: Dramatic New Evidence That Food Is Your Best Medicine* (New York: Bantam, 1988), 231–32.

9. *Bottom Line Health,* a wellness newsletter, carried this information in its August 1997 issue, p. 1, attributing to a report that appeared in *Cephalalgia,* a publication of the Henry Ford Hospital in Detroit.

10. Crayhon, 118.

11. *The PDR Family Guide to Nutrition and Health* (Montvale, NJ: Medical Economics, 1995), 233.

12. Winter and Winter, 58.

13. P. Geusens et al., "Long-Term Effect of Omega-3 Fatty Acid Supplementation in Active Rheumatoid Arthritis," *Arthritis and Rheumatism* 37, no. 6 (1994): 824–29.

14. M. A. Weiner and J. A. Weiner, *Herbs That Heal: Prescription for Herbal Healing* (Mill Valley, Calif.: Quantum Books, 1994) 39, 45, 46.

15. B. Gottlieb, *New Choices in Natural Healing* (Emmaus, Pa.: Rodale Press, 1995), 3.

16. Geoffrey Cowley, *Newsweek Interactive,* May 6, 1996.

17. S. J. Taussig et al., "Bromelain: A Proteolytic Enzyme and Its Clinical Application: A Review," *Hiroshima Journal of Medical Science* 24, nos. 2–3 (1975), 185–93.

18. M. Walker, "Non-Toxic Symptomatic Arthritis Relief Using Sea Cucumber (Beche-de-mer)," *Townsend Letter for Doctors* (October 1990), 1–6.

19. M. T. Murray, *The Healing Power of Herbs* (Rocklin, Calif.: Prima Publishing, 1993), 177.

Chapter 11: THE FUTURE OF MAGNET THERAPY

1. Preface, *Alternative Medicine: Expanding Medical Horizons.*

INDEX

acetaminophen, 84, 101–102, 103
acupuncture/acupressure, 21–22, 43,
  69, 93, 115
  magnet therapy compared to, com-
    bined with, 58, 70–73, 77,
    113–115, 123
  points illustrated, 116–121
Adderly, Brenda, 39–40, 62, 79, 184
Adey, W. Ross, 44, 67, 68
Aerospace Medicine, 64
aging, 159, 164, 165
  drug sensitivity, 98, 102, 103, 104,
    108
  exercise, 131–132, 138, 140, 142,
    145
  nutrition, 149, 169, 170
Agriculture, U.S. Dept. of, 160
alcohol, 103, 159–160, 166, 168,
  169
Alexander, F. M., 94
allergens, 161–162
American Journal of Acupuncture, 58
Ampère, André-Marie, 9
analgesics, 82, 95–109
  for acute vs. chronic pain, 87–88,
    89, 90
  analgesic effects of acupuncture,
    exercise, 71, 135–136
botanical, 175–178
headaches induced by, 83–84, 158
how they work, 96–97
narcotic, 87–89
  addiction to, 100, 105, 106–107
  opioid, 73, 89, 90, 92–93, 98,
    105–108
nonnarcotic, 92, 95–105
side effects, 95, 96, 99–108
use and overuse of, 6, 83, 88, 93,
  95–96, 108–109
antidepressants, 95, 98–99, 138,
  141–142, 147, 154, 167
antioxidants, 150, 159, 167, 169,
  170
  supplements, 163, 164, 165, 176
*Archives of Physical Medicine and Reha-
  bilitation*, 112
Ardito, G., 64
Aristotle, 22, 84
arthritis, 6, 87, 96
  diet/diet supplements and, 149,
    161–162, 174–175, 177, 178
  and exercise, 131, 132, 136–141
  magnet therapy for, 23, 37, 54, 61,
    137
  osteoarthritis, 96, 132, 136,
    140–141, 156, 169, 170

Arthritis, Rheumatism, and Aging
 Medical Information System, 96
Asclepius (god of healing), 175
ascorbic acid (Vitamin C), 100, 164,
 165, 169–170, 173
Ashmole, Elias, 25
aspirin, 99–100, 103, 104, 108
 and vitamin deficiency, 167, 169
Association for the Study of Pain, 43
Ayurvedic medicine, 177

back pain, 5–6, 82
 chronic, 89, 101, 107
 exercise and, 101, 107, 132–134,
  135, 138, 141
 magnet therapy for, 37, 98, 112
 psychological state and, 85, 89
 studies of, 132–133, 141, 160
 TENS therapy for, 92
Back Pain Association of America, 5
Bailly, Jean-Sylvain, 31
Barnothy, Madeleine F., 55–56
Baron, J. B., 59
battery, invention of, 32
Bayer Chemical Works, 99
B-complex vitamins, 165, 166–168
Becker, Robert O., 19, 38, 66–67, 68,
 72, 114
Bell's palsy, 74
beta-carotene, 149, 150, 164, 166
"Bioelectrical Applications in Medicine," 54
bioelectricity, 22
Bioelectromagnetics (journal), 57
Blakemore, Richard, 11
blood flow, 69, 70, 76, 113
blood sugar, blood glucose, 155, 157,
 160, 161
bone repair, 54, 57, 68
Bonita, John, 43
boswella, 177

brain stimulation, 73–75, 95, 150,
 171
British pain studies, 93–94, 160
bromelain, 176–177
Brown, Lonny J., 78
bursitis, 6, 37
Business Week, 69

caffeine, 83, 157–159, 167, 168
calcium, 157, 170–172, 173
Canada, NSAID use in, 101
cancer, 65, 68–71, 160
 diet and, 149, 150, 159, 169, 174
cancer cell destruction, 55–57, 64
Canon, James, 4
carbohydrates, 147, 155–156
carpal tunnel syndrome, 6, 168
 magnet therapy for, 37, 61, 112
Carper, Jean, 171
Celsus, Aulus Cornelius, 23–24
Chestnut, David, 4
Chicago World's Fair (1893), 35
Chinese medicine, 21, 22, 23, 43, 71,
 72, 175, 178
Christian Science movement, 34
chromium, dietary, 173–175
Cleopatra, 22
COAT (chronic opioid analgesic ther-
 apy), 106
coercivity, 16
Cohen, Leonardo G., 74
Colbert, Jim, 3, 62
copper, dietary, 173
Coy, Peter, 69
Cross Currents (Becker), 19, 66

Da Ponte, Lorenzo, 28
dehydration, 156, 157
dental surgery, 58
depression, 53, 68, 87, 132, 147, 168.
 See also antidepressants

Diogenes Laertius, 149
Driving Force (Livingston), 63
Duke University Medical Center, 85, 94

Eddy, Mary Baker, 34
EFAs (essential fatty acids), 153, 174–175
electrical pulse therapy, 92, 93
electricity, 9, 17, 22, 32
electromagnetism, 9, 11, 20, 35
   case for, 37, 46–48, 54, 55
   and health risk, 65–73
   pulsed, 14–15, 42, 45, 46, 51, 54, 65
   research on, 42–54
   See also magnetic fields (MF); magnet therapy
electromagnets, 12, 15–16, 17, 45
   compared to permanent magnets, *see* magnets, permanent
"electromedicine," 66, 68
Elizabeth I, queen of England, 26
EMS (eosinophilia myalgia syndrome), 154
end-gaining, 94
Eplin, Howard, 4
Euripides, 23
exercise, 130–146
   aerobic, 137–139, 140
   analgesic effect, 135–136
   as antidepressant, 140, 141–142
   and back pain, *see* back pain
   magnets used in conjunction with, 130, 132, 135, 137, 145, 146

Faraday, Michael, 9, 44, 72
fat, 147, 151–154, 171
   low-fat diet, *see* nutrition
feverfew, 178
fiber, 150–151. *See also* nutrition

fibrositis, fibromyalgia, 98, 132
"fight or flight," 162, 166
Finland studies, 132–133, 160
flavonoids, 150
Fleck, John, 132
folic acid (B-complex vitamin), 169
Food and Drug Administration (FDA), 37, 102, 112
Food Pharmacy, The (Carper), 171
For Your Health and Wealth magazine, 78
Franklin, Benjamin, 31, 33
free radicals, 164–165, 170, 173
French Academy of Science, 30, 32
French diet research, 152

Galvani, Luigi, 32
gate control theory, 91–92
Gauss, Carl Friedrich, 15, 32
gauss units, 15–17, 45, 55, 59, 61–65 *passim,* 76, 112
George, Mark, 53
German research, 72, 83, 172
Gilbert, William, 13, 25–26
ginger, 178
glucose and glycogen, 155–156
Golf Digest, 3
Göttingen Magnetic Union, 32
Greece, case study in, 49–51
Green, Arthur, 64
green drinks, 176
Guide to Alternative Medicine (Rosenfeld), 77
Guillotin, Joseph-Ignace, 31

Hall effect, 78
Hallett, Mark, 74
Halley, Edmund, 26, 31
Halpern, Myron H., 20, 64
Han, Kim Bong, 71
Hannemann, Holger, 20

headaches, 6, 83, 160, 172, 178
  analgesic-induced ("rebound"),
    83–84, 158
  chronic tension, 122, 134
  foods causing, 162
  magnet therapy for, 37, 81
Health & Healing newsletter, 184
heart disease, 132, 152, 159, 160
  vitamin E and, 170
Hell, Fr. Maximilian, 26–27
herbal medicine, 175–178
Hertz, Heinrich, 35
Hippocrates, 99
Hoffmann, Felix, 99
Holcomb, Robert, 77
Holmes, Steven, 60
Hopkins, Anthony, 4
Hospital Practice magazine, 5
Humboldt, Alexander von, 32

ibuprofen, 100–101
Indian medicine, 21, 22, 175, 177
inflammation, 37, 47, 70
  diet/diet supplements and, 147,
    153, 170, 174–178
  knee, *see* synovitis
  See also NSAIDs
insomnia, 68, 131, 154, 158–160
  passim, 168
Institutional Review Board, 112
International Association for the Study
  of Pain, 80
International Journal of Neuroscience,
  49, 75
ionization, 78
iron
  dietary, 147, 166, 172–173
  magnetism of, 12–13, 18, 19
iron oxides, 11, 13
Israeli study, 61, 76
Italy, analgesic use in, 83

Johns Hopkins University, 54
Journal of the American Medical Association, 74

Kahn, Joseph and Joyce, 4–5
Katz, Y. D., 53
Keeton, William, 11
Kennedy, Dr. and Mrs. Charles W. Jr.,
  111–112, 121
Kennedy, John F., 122
Kuz'menko, V. V., 53

Lafayette, Marquis de, 30
Lancet, The (medical journal), 161
Lavoisier, Antoine-Laurent, 31
Lawrence, Ronald, 43–44, 61, 62, 63,
  73, 69–70, 112
Lerchl, A., 75–76
leukemia, childhood, 65, 66, 69–71
levodopa therapy, 49–51
Linet, Martha S., 70
Livingston, James, 63
lodestone, 11, 13, 22, 23, 26, 71
Louis XVI, king of France, 31

McIndoe, Rosemary, 90, 131
McLean, M. J., 74
MAGNAflex Inc., 111–112
magnesium, 171, 172
Magnetic Company, 34–35
magnetic fields (MF), 9, 11, 14
  direction of, 17–18, 19
  electromagnetic, 70, 71, 74
  permanent, case for, 55–58
  pulsed, 14, 47, 54
  static, 14, 57, 71
  strength of (gauss), 15–17, 45
  within human body, 12, 19, 25
  See also electromagnetism
magnetic resonance imaging (MRI)
  machines, 15, 63

magnetism, 8–11, 19, 37–38
  "animal," 27–28, 30, 31, 34
  safety of, 65–67
  See also electromagnetism; magnetic
    fields (MF)
magnetite, 11
magnetoencephalogram (MEG), 19
magnets, permanent, 16, 58
  compared to electromagnets,
    14–15, 17, 44, 45–46, 55,
    74–75
  efficacy of, 42, 44–45, 46, 54,
    55–62, 74–75
  safety of, 15, 63–73, 74
  strength of (gauss units), 15–17, 45,
    76, 110
magnets, ubiquity of, 63. *See also* elec-
    tromagnets; magnets, permanent
magnet therapy
  acupuncture with, 113–115, 123
  acupuncture compared to, 58,
    70–73, 77
  advantages of, 112
  and blood flow, 69, 70, 76, 113
  devices for, 33, 34–35
  diet with, 7, 147
  difficulty in testing, 40–41
  drug therapy with, 108–109
  efficacy of, 5, 22, 42–62, 73, 76, 98,
    109, 111, 112
  electromagnetic, 15, 36, 42, 49–54,
    55, 75
  electromagnets vs. permanent mag-
    nets in, 14–15, 17, 44, 45-
    46, 55, 74–75
  exercise combined with, 7, 130,
    132, 135, 137, 145, 146
  future of, 180–184
  history of, 21–38
  how it works, 68–79
  how to use it, 110–123

levels of magnetism, 45–46
modern acceptance of, 37, 38
postoperative, 119
safety of, 7, 63–73, 74
  precautions, 72–73, 112–113
side effects, 48, 53, 64, 112–113
stress management along with, 7
Magnet Therapy (Hannemann), 20
Malthus, Thomas, 67
Maria Theresa, empress, 29
Marino, Dan, 3
Mashima, K., 141
maximum energy product, 16–17
Mediterranean diet, 152
Mehta, Jason, 163
melatonin, 54, 75, 76
Melzack, Ronald, 91, 115, 123
Mendyka, Edith, 132
menstrual pain, 6, 59–60
meridians, 21, 71–72, 114
Mesmer, Franz Anton, 26–32, 34, 36
Miami Dolphins, 3–4
migration, animal, 11
Milham, Samuel, 69
minerals/mineral supplements, 148,
    170–174
  recommended doses, 171–174
morphine, 92–93, 105–108 *passim*,
    114–115
Mozart, Wolfgang Amadeus, 28–29
Mueller, Robert, 124
Mulay, Indumati and L. N., 55
multiple sclerosis study, 51–52
myofascial pain. *See* pain

Nakagawa, Kyoichi, 5
National Academy of Science, 69–70
National Cancer Institute, 70
National Health Interview Survey, 87
National Institutes of Health, 53
Nature (British journal), 55, 64

neck pain study, 48–49

"neo" magnets, 13

New England Journal of Medicine, 71

Newsweek, 99

New York Times, 66

niacin, niacinamide (B3), 167

Nielsen, Arleigh, 4

Nobel Prize, 91

Nor, Fabio, 43

NSAIDs (nonsteroidal anti-inflammatory drugs), 92, 95–105, 109, 141. *See also* analgesics

nutrition, 147–162, 179
 diet supplements, 163–178
 items to limit or avoid, 157–162
 low-fat, high-carbohydrate diet, 148–151, 153, 154
 Mediterranean diet, 152
 plant foods, 148–151, 153, 171
 studies of, 152, 161–162

Oersted, Hans Christian, 9

omega oils, 153, 174–175

opiate/opioid drugs, 89, 90, 98, 105–108
 endogenous peptides, 73, 92–93

"opium poppy," 105, 175

orgone energy accumulator, 36–37

Ornish, Dean, 152

osteoporosis, 132, 140, 157, 171–172

osteopuncture, 43

oxidation. *See* antioxidants

Pace, Adele, 130

pain
 acute vs. chronic, 87–90, 92, 93
 allergies and, 161–162
 definitions of, 80–81, 88–89
 emotional factors in, 94
 exercise and, 101, 106, 132–136, 138, 140–142, 145

gate control theory, 91–92
 as "learned experience," 86
 prevalence of, 6, 84, 182
 reaction to/threshold of, 81–83, 85–86, 89–90, 93–94, 136, 174
 referred (myofascial), 88, 92, 115, 122–123
 studies of, 82, 85, 93–94, 132–133, 141, 160
 See also back pain; headaches

painkillers. *See* analgesics

Palmer, Daniel, 34

Panminerva Med (journal), 47

pantothenic acid (B5), 167–168

Paracelsus, 23–25, 27

Parkinson's disease study, 49–51

Peikert, Andreas, 172

Perkins, Elisha, 33

Pert, Candace, 92

Philostratus, 139

phlogistic process defined, 47

Physical Therapy Forum, 4

phytochemicals, 149–150, 166

pineal gland, 54, 75–76

placebo effect, 40, 42, 48, 52, 62, 82, 114
 Johns Hopkins study of, 54

plant foods. *See* nutrition

Plato, 22

potassium, 100, 172

power lines, 65, 68, 71

pregnancy, 72, 112, 159, 178

Prince, Jack P., 52

protein, 147, 151, 168

psychological factors, 89, 90, 93–94, 131

pyridoxine (B6), 168

qi (*ch'i* or *chi*), 21–22

Quen, Jacques, 33

Quimby, Phineas, 34

Rabinovich, E. Z., 60
Radner, Gilda, 66
Raylman, Raymond, 57
Reich, Wilhelm, 36–37
Reichmanis, Maria, 114
Reuters news service, 96
riboflavin (B2), 167
Rosenfeld, Isadore, 83
Russian research, 53–54, 60

Salk Institute, 70
Sandyk, Reuven, 49, 51, 52, 81
Sanseverino, Riva, 46, 75
saturation magnetization, 16–17
sciatica, 6, 89, 160

Sears, Roebuck and Company, 34
selenium, 174
serotonin, 75, 76, 99, 147, 154, 168
SIA (stimulation-induced analgesia), 95
sinter, 13–14
sleeping pills, 168, 169
smoking, 160
soft tissue damage, 54, 60, 68, 140
South African study of NSAIDs, 141
space program, U.S., 20
stair climbing, 138–139
Stepanov, E. A., 60
Stevens, Charles, 70
strength training, 140–142
stress-related disorders, 68, 87, 89
stretching, 142–144
Sturgeon, William, 12
sugar, 160, 161
Surgeon General's Report, 131
Swedish pain studies, 85, 141
swimming, 138. *See also* exercise

Swiss pain study, 85
synovitis, 61, 76, 112

Tata, D. B., 56–57
TENS (transcutaneous electrical nerve stimulation), 92, 93, 95, 157–158
Tesla, Nikola, 35
Thacher, C. J., 34–35
Thailand headache clinic, 83
thiamine (B1), 157, 166–167
Thomas, Keith, 25
transdermal drug delivery system (patches), 113
Travell, Janet, 122
trigger points, 122–123, 124–129
tryptophan, 147, 151, 154, 167, 171
turmeric, 183–184

ulcer complications (as NSAID side effect), 96, 101, 103, 104
University of Manitoba, 58
University of Texas, 82
University of Tokyo, 77
University of Washington, 43
urethral stenosis study, 60

Vandyk, J. H., 20
vasodilation. *See* blood flow
vegetables. *See* nutrition
vegetarians, 149, 169
Veterans Administration, 132
vitamins, 148, 153, 165–171
    excretion of, 100, 157
    supplements, 150, 166–173
Volta, Alessandro, 32

Wall, Patrick, 91
Washington, George, 30
water, body's need for, 156

INDEX

Weber, Wilhelm, 32
Weinberger, A., 82
Weissler, Vicki, 116
Whitaker, Julian, 110, 148, 152, 164, 170, 173, 184
Whitaker Wellness Institute, 110
Winter, Arthur, 155

women, 82, 85, 94, 103, 131
World Health Organization, 65

yin and yang, 21

zinc, dietary, 173